PLANT SCIENCE RESEARCH AND PRACTICES

NATURAL ANTI-AGING PLANTS AND DELAY OF SENESCENCE

Plant Science Research and Practices

Additional books and e-books in this series can be found on Nova's website under the Series tab.

New Developments in Medical Research

Additional books and e-books in this series can be found on Nova's website under the Series tab.

PLANT SCIENCE RESEARCH AND PRACTICES

NATURAL ANTI-AGING PLANTS AND DELAY OF SENESCENCE

NOBORU MOTOHASHI
EDITOR

nova
Medicine & Health
New York

NOTICE TO THE READER

Library of Congress Cataloging-in-Publication Data

Names: Motohashi, Noboru, editor.
Title: Natural anti-aging plants and delay of senescence / Noboru Motohashi, editor.
Other titles: Plant science research and practices.
Description: [Hauppauge, N.Y.] : Nova Science Publishers, [2019] | Series: Plant science research and practices | Includes bibliographical references and index. |
Identifiers: LCCN 2019041484 (print) | LCCN 2019041485 (ebook) | ISBN 9781536162820 (paperback) | ISBN 9781536162837 (adobe pdf)
Subjects: LCSH: Materia medica, Vegetable. | Aging--Prevention.
Classification: LCC RS164 .N33 2019 (print) | LCC RS164 (ebook) | DDC 612.6/7--dc23
LC record available at https://lccn.loc.gov/2019041484
LC ebook record available at https://lccn.loc.gov/2019041485

Published by Nova Science Publishers, Inc. † New York

CONTENTS

PREFACE

Humans have a strong desire to health and complete their lives from birth to death. Furthermore, it is natural that humans want to live long life and have few diseases. This is the greatest happiness of human beings. The nutrition of pregnant women has been thought to affect the health of the fetus, neonates, adults and even the elderly. Ultimately, mother's nutritional status in the fetus is considered to be one of the causes that affect human's future health. So we can understand how the nutritional support of pregnant women is important for the healthy development of the fetus.

Since ancient times, the region-specific folklore remedies such as Ayurveda and Chinese Traditional Medicine (CTM) have been used throughout the world. Human used different plants to treat common and many deadly diseases. They are familiar with the uses of plants that are available to medicinal plants in nature. According to the World Health Organization (WHO), cancer and diabetes are the most deadly diseases in the world. To date, traditional treatments for medicine have been actively prescribed, and about 80% of the world's population use plants to treat common diseases. Diabetes, which is a lifestyle-related disease, has the potential to cause various diseases by raising blood sugar levels. In general, plant-derived drug formulations cause few side effects in the human body. Plants are one of the antioxidant natural materials such as antioxidants, flavonoids, tannins and vitamin C. They control the function of β-cells and are effective in regulating blood sugar levels. The use of herbal medicines is a great attempt to prevent and treat chronic diseases. Plant-based prescription drugs are highly safe and inexpensive. For this reason, diabetes treatment can be expected to establish more effective prevention and treatment methods through new trials such as herbal medicine combinations.

Cocoa seeds are effective in improving dementia and delaying aging. The main medicinal effects of these anti-aging results from the bioavailability and metabolism of antioxidants. In recent years, with the increasing trend of the longevity population worldwide, interest related to aging and aging is increasing. This age-related lifestyle-related disease is a decline in physical activity and quality of life, and a human pathological risk factor. Healthy aging is associated with an excellent nutritional balance and an increase in the modest intake of bioactive compounds such as the antioxidant component flavonoid. The beneficial effects of age-related cocoa flavonoids are that consumption of cocoa flavonoids prolongs the life of old rats and manifests a reduction in mortality in diabetic mice. Furthermore, this effect induces cranial nerve development in the hippocampus etc. and works to enhance cognitive ability. Individuals who consume large amounts of cacao from their daily diet have shown lower incidence such as diabetes, ischemic heart disease, and stroke, and significantly longer lifespan, when compared to low cacao consumers. However, as people reduced their consumption of cacao, these beneficial effects disappeared. Therefore, dietary supplementation with cacao flavonoids and their long-term intake can be expected to ameliorate age-related problems and some cognitive disorders.

With age, humans begin to decrease sex hormones and other hormone secretions. Decreased hormone secretion tends to cause lifestyle-related diseases such as diabetes, brain disease (Parkinson's disease and Alzheimer's disease), hypertension, heart failure, eye strain, diabetes, various cancers, neuralgia and other visceral diseases. Therefore, humans should supply the reduced amounts of hormones to avoid these diseases.

Chapter 1 - Fetal malnutrition derived from pregnant women is a factor that greatly affects the health status of not only the mother but also the fetus and the offspring. According to the epidemiological survey, it suggests that postnatal infants and adults with poor fetal nutrition may even have an impact on disease resistance and lifespan. For example, protein intake during the diet of a pregnant woman is one of the very important factors in determining the general physical condition of an infant at birth. Thus, according to epidemiological surveys, proteins are widely involved in pregnancy diets, such as height at birth, birth weight, and general physical health condition of infants at birth. The semiessential amino acid L-arginine (L-Arg. **5**) is one of the amino acids that is particularly expected in the field of chemotherapy such as prevention and treatment of lifestyle-related diseases by improving active oxygen nitric oxide (NO) formation. Peroxisome proliferator-activated receptor gamma (γ) coactivator 1α (PGC-1α) plays an important role in the regulation of many genes that affects a wide range of physiological functions, due to its interaction with other signaling pathways that control mitochondrial homeostasis and protein balance. Aging is a negative factor for PGC-1α gene expression. Thus, increasing stimulation of this pathway through age-related diseases can maintain and enhance PGC-1α signaling activity and then improve the related functions at the site of aging. In order to maintain the health of mothers, fetuses and adults, it is suggested that mothers should have a well-balanced diet before and after pregnancy.

Chapter 2 - In later days of twentieth century, use of plant/plant products as medicine has attracted the attention of a large number of population and also the scientific community. It helped to expand the use of herbs to treat the ailment. Medicinal plants have been the main source of the traditional as well as the modern medicinal therapy. Use of phytochemicals is economically viable and easily available resource. The history reveals that Chinese used plants as medicine firstly and India followed it later. Later on, ancient general practitioners have studied the properties and therapeutic uses of plants of medicinal importance. Thus, it has been developed as indigenous system of medicine which became a fundamental platform in India for the primordial medical discipline. In most of the developing countries, a large number of people mainly depend on traditional methods to address their health issues. In spite of great development in the modern medicinal therapy, traditional remedy and herbal medicines have sustained their esteem for historic and intellectual basis. In recent years, applying the information of herbs in modern medicinal remedies has gained interest around the world due to their significant effects on health issues. Products of plant have played vital function in the prevention and treatment of many diseases all over the globe. This has compelled the scientists to gather information on traditional remedy that makes use of phytochemicals. There are a wide range of resources containing bioactive contents available on the planet. Almost all the plant sources possesses significant properties which are beneficiary in solving the health issues. Plants may possess antioxidant, antibacterial, antimicrobial, antifungal, anticancer, antidiabetic, antihyperlipidemic, antihyperlipidemic, anti-inflammatory, antiviral, antiaging, and other activities. It is estimated that almost 50-60 % of patients with different types of cancer consume drugs which are isolated from various plants and/or their products. It is being utilized as complementary to chemotherapy and/or radiation therapy. Less side effects are reported for phytochemicals as drugs. In view of this, natural components of plant sources can be practiced for the effective and natural treatment of diseases like cancer and diabetes.

Chapter 3 - *Theobroma cacao* is a tropical tree of Sterculiaceae family. The cacao seeds are economically important because they are used to elaborate chocolate. Pre-Columbian civilizations consumed cacao seeds and some derived products due to its medicinal attributes (build up resistance and fights fatigue). The purpose of this Chapter is essentially to describe and highlight on the main flavonoids present in cacao and their applications on cognitive health and senescence. It is well known that a rich diet in flavonoids improved health condition. Moreover, these beneficial effects depend on the flavonoids bioavailability and metabolism, mediated by flavonoids´ stereochemistry, flavonoid-flavonoid interaction, flavonoid-food matrix interaction and flavonoid-gut microbiota interaction. During flavonoids metabolism monomers are degraded faster than oligomers. Aging and senescence´s related problems are increasing worldwide, and this deterioration not only results in reduced physical activity and quality of life, but also is the primary risk factor for human pathologies. Healthy aging has been related to lifestyle, good nutrient balance and to a higher intake of bioactive compounds such as flavonoids. The age-related beneficial effect of cacao flavonoids, has been studied in preclinical models and in clinical trials. These studies reported that consumption of cacao flavonoids might increase lifespan in aged rats, reduced mortality of diabetic mice, induced neurogenesis in the hippocampus and subventricular zone of adult mice and improved cognitive performance. Moreover, a study on the San Blas Island population, which consume high quantities of cacao showed lower incidence of diabetes, ischemic heart disease, stroke and a remarkably longer lifespan. However, these beneficial effects disappeared when people reduce their cacao consumption. Thus, diet supplementation with cacao flavonoids and its long term intake can improve aged related problems and some cognitive diseases.

Chapter 4 - In general, diseases associated with aging are inevitable diseases for humans which are involved in the entire body such as cardiovascular system (heart disease), respiratory system (pneumonia), digestive system (reflux esophagitis), kidney and urinary system (incontinence), nervous system (Alzheimer's disease, Parkinson's disease), bone and motor system (osteoporosis), sensory organ system (senile cataract), degradation of masticatory forces and so on. Humans will need some treatment for these diseases with age. The reason for this is that elderly people are more likely to suffer from physiological dysfunction with age than young people. Humans must minimize this physiological dysfunction in order to stay fit for the rest of their lives. As humans age, their hormonal performance may decline, and sometimes even increase, as compared to their younger age. Therefore, humans need to re-set their normal hormone balance, that is, homeostasis (hormone homeostasis), with normal hormone balance, that is, the symptoms associated with insufficient secretion or increased secretion of hormones, or imbalance or increase in hormone balance involved in most important physiological functions.

Proper hormonal treatment is thought to regulate, stop or delay changes in hormone production with age. Therefore, in this Chapter, we mainly described to the representative human growth hormone (HGH), melatonin, thyrotropin, thyroid hormone, calcitonin (CT), dehydroepiandrosterone (DHEA), aldosterone, and estrogen that are currently expected for hormone therapy, and described based on their effects on the physiological functions and the results of epidemiological surveys of each hormone.

Noboru Motohashi, PhD
Foreign Examiner for Evaluation of the PhD Thesis in Indian National University, India and Former Professor and Director (elected Riji in Japanese) of *Meiji Pharmaceutical University*, Tokyo Japan
E-mail: noborumotohashi@jcom.home.ne.jp

May 16, 2019

In: Natural Anti-Aging Plants …
Editor: Noboru Motohashi
ISBN: 978-1-53616-282-0

Chapter 1

RELATIONSHIP BETWEEN NUTRITION DURING PREGNANCY AND SENESCENCE

***Noboru Motohashi*[1,*], *Anuradha Vanam*[2,†], *Jyothirmayi Vadapalli*[3,‡] and *Rao Gollapudi*[4,§]**
[1]Meiji Pharmaceutical University, Kiyose-shi, Tokyo, Japan
[2]Sri Venkateswara University, Tirupathi, AP, India
[3]Acharya Nagarjuna University, Nagarjunanagar, AP, India
[4]University of Kansas, Lawrence, Kansas, US

ABSTRACT

Fetal malnutrition (fetal nutrition disorder) derived from pregnant women is a factor that greatly affects the health status of not only the mother but also the fetus and the offspring. According to the epidemiological survey, it suggests that postnatal infants and adults with poor fetal nutrition may even have an impact on disease resistance and lifespan. For example, protein intake of a pregnant woman is one of the

* Corresponding Author's E-mail: noborumotohashi@jcom.home.ne.jp.
† Corresponding Author's E-mail: agollapdr@gmail.com.
‡ Corresponding Author's E-mail: jyothi.galactica@gmail.com.
§ Corresponding Author's E-mail: gollapudirao@ku.edu.

very important factors in determining the general physical condition of an infant at birth. Thus, according to epidemiological surveys, proteins are widely involved in pregnancy diets, such as height at birth, birth weight, and general physical health condition of infants at birth.

The semiessential amino acid L-arginine (L-Arg. 5) is one of the amino acids that are adjuvantly applied in the field of chemotherapy including prevention and treatment of lifestyle-related diseases by improving active nitric oxide (NO) formation.

Peroxisome proliferator-activated receptor gamma (γ) coactivator 1α (PGC-1α) plays an important role in the regulation of many genes that affects a wide range of physiological functions, due to its interaction with other signaling pathways that control mitochondrial homeostasis and protein balance. Aging is a negative factor for PGC-1α gene expression. Thus, increasing stimulation of this pathway through age-related diseases can maintain and enhance PGC-1α signaling activity and then improve the related functions at the site of aging.

In order to maintain the health of mothers, fetuses and adults, it is suggested that mothers should have a well-balanced diet before and after pregnancy.

Keywords: aging, senescence, *Dutch famine*, arginine paradox, PGC-1α

Chemical Constituents in Antiaging

riboflavin (vitamin B2. **1**)
thiamine (vitamin B1. **2**)
niacin (vitamin B3. nicotinic acid. **3**)
ascorbic acid (vitamin C. **4**)
L-arginine (L-Arg. **5**)
rapamycin (**6**)

Abbreviations

AIDS	acquired immune deficiency syndrome
CC	correlation coefficient
cDNA	complementary DNA

CNS	central nervous system
CP	cerebral infantile palsy (cerebral palsy)
E. coli	*Escherichia coli*
GOE	great oxygenation event
HIV	human immunodeficiency virus
IlS	insulin/insulin-like growth factor (IGF) signaling
hsp	*heat shock protein*
IGF	insulin/insulin-like growth factor
MHC	myosin heavy chain
MRP	mammalian protei
MRPs	mitochondrial ribosomal proteins
mtDNA	mitochondrial DNA
nDNA	nuclear DNA
NO	nitric oxide
NRC	the National Research Council
NRF	nuclear respiratory factor
NTDs	*neglected tropical diseases*
OXPHOS	oxidative phosphorylation
PGC-1α)	proliferator-activated receptor gamma (γ) coactivator 1α
PKU	phenylketonuria
PPARγ or PPARG	peroxisome proliferator-activated receptor gamma
ROS	reactive oxygen species
rRNAs	ribosomal RNAs
SE	standard error
sod	*superoxide dismutase*
tRNAs	transfer RNAs
TOR	target of rapamycin
UCP1	uncoupling protein-1
WWII	World War II

1. INTRODUCTION

1.1. On the Birth of Life and Death

Living organisms, including humans, have been going through birth and death processes. First, according to life origin theory of *abiogenesis, or informally the origin of life*, the birth of life is the process of conversion to the body (life form or the life organism) characterized by life-like organisms such as self-proliferation ability, energy conversion ability and homeostatic preservation from inanimate objects such as simple organisms. In theory the living form is produced from inorganic matter. In the primitive earth which was born approximately 4.4 billion years ago, photosynthesis by cyanobacteria (stromatolite which is still present as a spherical or cylindrical coalite fossil with a lamina-like structure made by algae) took place since 3 billion years to about 1 billion years ago on introduction of free oxygen into the atmosphere, great oxygenation event (GOE) and oxygen crisis [1, 2, 3, 4]. Consequently, a large number of abiotic organic matters made from extremely limited elements such as hydrogen, nitrogen, and oxygen in the atmosphere gathers and coalesces into *a droplet shape* with no membrane in the sea. *Droplets* with a baglike structure have acquired life forms over a long period of time and evolved into nerve cell bodies of neurons in which nuclei are present in neurons (neurons). However, in addition to the *theory of droplet*, various theories are argued in the theory of life origin [1, 2, 3, 4].

Second, in 2010, MIT magazine posted "All living things must be aged and die?" In the process of evolution, even though immortality is possible; it would not be desirable to manipulate the organism. From ageing, and ultimately to death, the result is accumulation of damage to the organism over time. There is exhaustion of DNA due to the exposure to chemicals in the environment, radiation, or copy error where cells may not divide correctly, proteins may accidentally collapse, tissue may gradually deteriorate, or catastrophic disease or system outage may occur. Nevertheless, this regrettable advance called aging has logic. The aging strategy, which seems to be used by nature many times, is to kill the cells and organisms that have accumulated all such damage, and conquer the descendants of the new world.

While evolution prefers death, it is thought that there is no theoretical reason why an organism could not evolve into immortality. For example, Gram-positive radiation resistant bacteria *Deinococcus radiodurans* can survive even under severe radiation damage and extreme cold acidic conditions. In addition, a small invertebrate beetle Tardigrades with a length of about 1 mm seems not to be affected by long-term dehydration, heat, and even the vacuum of the universe.

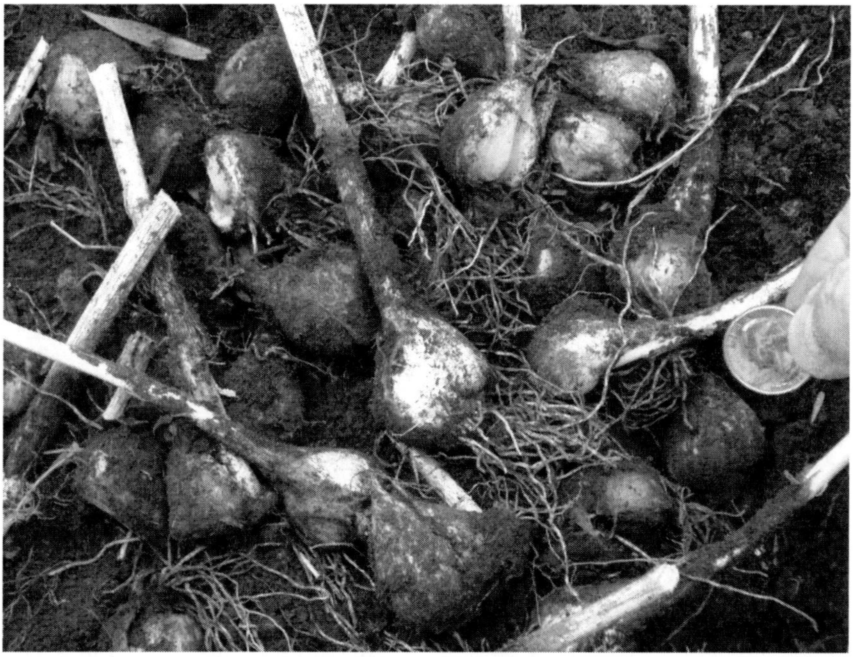

Photo 1. Garlic (*Allium sativum*) at home garden of author Noboru Motohashi in Tokyo. Photographed by Noboru Motohashi. 8/8/2008 Fri.

Humans probably will not completely conquer the death. However, human life spans have risen rapidly for centuries, at least in developed areas of the world. Subsequently, further research will prolong longevity to humans. Recent studies have confirmed the possibility of retarding the aging and lifestyle diseases in many organisms, as foods close to starvation modify the activity of specific proteins. Aging related researchers are looking for antiaging foods (garlic) (Photo 1) and other antiaging compounds that can be healthy and delay aging for at least a long period of time.

However, the dangers associated with this dream alchemy medicine (panacea) are hidden. Humans trying to escape from death and disease may still have age-related changes with regard to their own ideas and reactions to diseases. These anti-aging compounds can also prevent certain diseases by interfering with essential biological processes; however, there is also the possibility of developing or accelerating another new disease [5].

2. Delay of Senescence

2.1. Human Life and Death

It is suggested that about half of all deaths among 40-year-olds and three-fourths of 50-year-olds in USA resulted from aging since 1999 and 2015 [6, 7].

Depending on the mortality experience in 2016 in USA, first, a total of 2,744,248 resident deaths were registered in USA, yielding a crude death rate of 849.3 in 100,000 populace. Second, the age-adjusted death rate, which accounts for the aging of the population, was 728.8 deaths in 100,000 populace. Third, life expectancy at birth was 78.6 years.

Fourth, among the 15 main leading causes of deaths (total death number a) in 2016, heart disease (23.1%) is the highest, followed by malignant neoplasms (cancer)(21.8%); accidents (unintentional injuries)(5.9%); chronic lower respiratory diseases (chronic lower respiratory tract infection is a disease in which local infection defense ability is lowered and persistent bacterial infection is recognized because it has a basic disease in the airway below the tracheal bifurcation where no bacteria normally exist.) (5.6%); cerebrovascular diseases (stroke)(5.2%); Alzheimer's disease (AD) (4.2%); diabetes mellitus (DM) (2.9%); influenza & pneumonia(1.9%); nephritis, nephrotic syndrome and nephrosis (kidney disease)(1.8%); intentional self-harm (suicide)(1.6%); septicemia(1.5%); chronic liver disease and cirrhosis(1.5%); essential hypertension & hypertensive renal disease (hypertension) (1.2%); Parkinson's disease(1.1%); pneumonitis due to solids & liquids(0.7%); and all other causes (residual)(19.9%), respectively [7, 8].

2.2. What Is Aging?

In 1978, Dr. Comfort A. defined aging as follows: human aging is presumed to be caused by a wide range of environmental stresses to humans and their cumulative accumulation that continues throughout the life [9].

Moreover, genetic fitness components as two main qualifiers were added to Dr. Comfort's 1991 definition. According to Hamilton's law, aging has been considered to be a reduction or disappearance (out-of-step) of adaptation with increasing age by momentarily declining the power of natural selection.

This means that the first is a continuous fitness-component decline, whereas the second is a decline in physiological function. Therefore, senescence also occurs in the cells that make up the body's organs. A decrease in the number of cells and their function will also cause a decrease in functions of organs. Due to the decrease in body water content, dehydration may also cause deterioration of organ function [10, 11]. Thus, the increases in mortality with age due to chronic infections such as human immunodeficiency virus (HIV)/acquired immune deficiency syndrome (AIDS) were removed from the 1991 definition [10, 12].

In 2013, aging is characterized by *molecular denaturation* such as reduction of telomere length, genomic instability, and epigenetic alterations, *loss of proteostasis*, *deregulated nutrient sensing*, *cellular senescence* such as deregulated signaling, and mitochondrial dysfunction, *stem cell exhaustion*, *physiologic denaturation* such as inflammation, and insulin sensitivity, *functional alteration* such as sensory, balance, physical strength and ability, cognitive, cardiovascular functions, *altered intercellular communication*, and *life style-related diseases* such as heart disease, Alzheimer's disease, diabetes, cancer, osteoporosis. Therefore, aging is considered to be involving these comprehensive diseases with nonlinear pleiotropic characteristics [13, 14].

2.3. The Relationship between Fetal Undernutrition (Fetal Malnutrition) and Increased Risk of Metabolic Disease Later in Life (Relationship between Fetal Malnutrition and Life Expectancy)

In the second session, Dr. Janet King of Children's Hospital Oakland Research Institute emphasized the strong connection between in-utero nutrition and its outcomes later in life. Much of the early evidence for this connection comes from studies on the Dutch famine during World War II and from Dr. David Barker's analyses of 1920s data collected in England and Wales.

2.3.1. Influence of Prenatal Diet on the Mother and Child

Generally, apart from congenital abnormalities such as brain anoxia of endogenous anoxia brain fever, both birth traumas (birth injuries of the newborn) such as brachial plexus palsy, caput succedaneum, cephalhematoma, subgaleal hemorrhage, linear skull fracture, depressed skull fracture, subdural hematoma and traumatic intracerebral hematoma, and prematurity are unexplainable deaths [15].

Based on these facts, in 1942, a group of Departments of Paediatrics and Obstetrics, University of Toronto, Canada examined the influence of prenatal diet on the mother and child. First, patients were classified into three diet groups as follows: patients receiving *a poor diet throughout (Poor Diet Group. G1)*, patients on *dietary supplemented diet (Supplemented-Good Group. G2)*, and patients subsisting on *a good healthy diet* and receiving *advice (Good Diet Group. G3)*.

Second, nutritive factors (per day) by the recommended Good Diet used in this study were as follows: calories (2400-2,800); protein (80-100 g); fat (80-100 g); carbohydrate (350-400 g); calcium (1.5 g); iron (0.020 g); iodine (in iodized salt); vitamins: A (6,000 International Units (I.U.)), B1 (500-1000 I.U.), B2 (3.0-3.5 mg), C (50-75 mg), D (500-1000 I.U.), respectively.

Third, on the observations related to pregnancy, the past obstetrician history (per cent (%) of cases) of multiple pregnant patients are 71.4 (*G1*), 68.7 (*G2*), and 48.9 (*G3*), respectively. The breakdown of each case of multiple pregnancy patients in these three groups (*G1, G2, G3*) was as follows: 13.1 (*G1*), 4.7 (*G2*), and 9.0 (*G3*) for abortions; 38.1 (*G1*), 39.0 (*G2*), and 24.4 (*G3*) for miscarriages; 10.7 (*G1*), 20.3 (*G2*), and 13.3 (*G3*) for premature birth; 9.5 (*G1*), and 4.7 (*G2*), and 2.2 (*G3*) for stillbirths, respectively. Three per cent of the patients in *G3* had also ingested other sources such as extra milk, meat, vegetables, and fruits in addition to the recommended Good Diet. In addition, the same three per cent of the patients in the *G3* could participate as the group improved by education. The past obstetrical records of the multiparous patients showed a much higher incidence of previous major complications in *G1* and *G2* when compared to that (incidence of major complications) of *G3*.

Fourth, regarding ~~to~~ the relation between prenatal diet and the disease onset by breast milk malnutrition, principal illnesses in infants during first six months (per cent of cases) were as follows: 21.0 (*G1*), 4.7 (*G2*), and 4.7 (*G3*) for easiness of colds; 4.2 (*G1*), 1.5 (*G2*), and 5.7 (*G3*) for bronchitis; 5.5 (*G1*), 1.5 (*G2*), and 0.9 (*G3*) for pneumonia; 5.5 (*G1*), 0 (*G2*), and 0.9 (*G3*) for rickets; 4.2 (*G1*), 0 (*G2*), and 0 (*G3*) for tetany; 7.0 (*G1*), 1.5 (*G2*), and 0 (*G3*) for dystrophy; 25.0 (*G1*), 9.4 (*G2*), and 17.1 (*G3*) for anemia; 3 (*G1*), 0 (*G2*), and 0 (*G3*) for deaths, respectively.

From above result, a brief summary can be given of the first 250 infants followed to the age of six months. The increase of incidence on both minor diseases and major diseases in the infants born to the mothers in *G1* is more remarkable when compared to that (incidence) of *G2* or *G3*. The total general health condition of infants in *G2* was much better when compared to that (general health condition) of *G1* or *G3*. The mother's diet can be implied significantly by looking at the health condition of infants.

Two of the three infant deaths in *G1* resulted from pneumonia, whereas prematurity was the third cause of death.

From results mentioned above, the prenatal diets of 400 women with low incomes were studied. *First*, regarding the relationship between alimentation and prenatal diets, *one group (G1*) with a poor diet was treated as a control. *A second group (G2)* on a poor diet was improved by supplying food during the last three or four months of pregnancy. *A third group (G3)* with moderately good prenatal diets was improved by dietary counselling alone.

Second, the incidence of miscarriages, stillbirths, and premature births in poor diet group (*G1*) was much increased when compared to that (incidence) of *G2* and *G3*.

Third, the incidence of illness in the infants up to the age of six months and the number of deaths resulting from these illnesses were many times greater in *G1* when compared to that (incidence) of *G2* and *G3*.

Until today, it has been thought that there are many important factors in normal pregnancy and infant health. As a conclusion, this study suggests the following: Maternal nutrition during pregnancy at fetal stage has a major influence on the entire course of the fetus. In addition, fetal maternal nutrition markedly affects infant health during the first 6 months of birth [15, 16].

2.3.2. Importance of Pregnant Diet for Both Mother and Infant

Among the nutrients necessary for human growth, protein is a very vital nutrient and it is also one of the three major nutrients. In addition, it is essential for growth factors as protein not only supplies the necessary amount corresponding to the age in human growth period but also the good quality protein as a source of the essential amino acid indispensable for human growth that must be contained in the meal itself. It is known that particularly last two trimesters (total 6 months) of pregnancy is the period of rapid fetal growth and development. Therefore, an increase in the amount of protein in the pregnant woman's meal is essential during the last *two* trimester periods. However, many obstetricians usually did not inform the importance of the last *two* trimesters to pregnant women.

In 1939, Dr. Sronacar JR administered different proteins in rat feed in rat diet through six generations in order to investigate the effect of various levels of protein intake at reproductive time on the growth and development of offspring. As a result, the optimal protein dose to rats was a protein that accounted for around 14% of the total calorie of the diet. According to studies of optimal protein balance over six generations of rats, healthy rats are endowed with abundant protein balanced diet. Therefore, it is suggested that approximately 14% of the total calorie dietary protein has taken over continuity of healthy rats through generations, resulting in increased proteins into the rat body through efficient enzyme metabolism and the like [17].

In 1942, it is found that in latter pregnancy period, the pregnant mother organs store nitrogen in excess of nitrogen going into the developing fetus [18].

In both 1930 and 1934, it has been also confirmed that nitrogen retention in pregnant women was highest when sufficient animal protein was supplied during pregnant women's diet [19, 20].

Further, nitrogen retention in the fetus of each month during pregnancy was examined. As a result, the fetus has a protein requirement of about 845-900 g per day. Therefore, this protein demand per day is essential to maintain the above protein requirement as one indication of the total requirement including the fetus and accompanying minor organization structure during pregnancy [17]. These studies also suggested that pregnant women held 200 to 400 g of nitrogen per day in their bodies under the favorable environment. For the purpose of maintaining 200-400 g of nitrogen per day during pregnancy, pregnant women must maintain and supply body protein (1,250-2,500 g) constituting the body by each meal. These body protein supplements require a body protein increase of roughly 10-20 g in the last six months of pregnancy when compared to the daily required amount of regular daily women. These metabolic studies show the necessity of high protein intake during the last trimester of pregnancy. However, the effects of different body protein levels have little impact in the performance of pregnancy.

Moreover, in 1943, there was an apparent relationship between the mother's diet (mean general rating) during pregnancy, & the condition of the infant at birth and during the first two weeks of life, by using 216 mothers and their infants [21]. Besides, it was confirmed that the amount of protein ingested from the meal during pregnancy period greatly influences these correlations.

Based on the above facts, in 1943, a group of Department of Child Hygiene, Harvard School of Public Health, Boston, Mass. USA examined the importance of diet during pregnancy to both the mother and her infant. Different effects of maternal protein intake on infant's condition at birth were epidemiologically examined by grouping 216 mother's meals based on the average protein content in latter pregnancy period.

First, regarding the daily estimated dietary intake of protein in the mother's meal from 4 months to 9 months pregnancy, these results were *Excellent* (protein 85 or more, number of cases: 22; percentage of cases: 10%); *Good* (protein 70-84 g, number of cases: 47; percentage of cases: 22%); *Fair* (protein 55-69 g, number of cases: 66; percentage of cases: 30%); *Poor* (protein 45-54 g, number of cases: 51; percentage of cases: 24%); and *Very poor* (less than protein 45 g, number of cases: 30; percentage of cases: 14%), respectively.

According to the daily estimated dietary intake, only 10% of pregnant women are presumed to be *Excellent* with regard to proteins. Contrary to this, 68% of pregnant women had taken less than *Fair* meal.

Second, on the relationship between the amount of protein in pregnant women 's diet and body height at the birth of an infant, average protein intake per day for pregnant women and body height at the birth of infant were follows: *Excellent* (protein: 85 g or more; number of infant (boys): 10; mean length at birth: 53.3 cm)/(girls): 10; mean length at birth: 52.0 cm); *Good* (protein: 70-84 g; number of infant (boys): 21; mean length at birth: 51.4 cm)/(girls) : 22; mean length at birth: 51.0 cm); *Fair* (protein: 55-69 g; number of infant (boys): 29; mean length at birth: 50.3 cm)/(girls) : 32; mean length at birth: 49.9 cm); *Poor* (protein: 45-54 g; number of infant (boys): 25; mean length at birth: 49.3 cm)/(girls) : 21; mean length at birth: 48.7 cm); *Very poor* (protein: under 45 g; number of infant (boys): 7; mean length at birth: 47.4 cm)/(girls) : 8; mean length at birth: 46.6 cm), respectively.

Third, the percentile criteria (percentile value) of the body height and body weight of infants in the full-term birth (births between the 37th week and the 41th week of gestation) were examined. Since actual differences exist between the body height and body weight of male or female infants at birth, the height and weight of each infant was expressed as a percentile range.

Body height (cm) and body weight (pound) at the time of boy's (or girl's) birth were the tenth infant out of 100: 48.1 cm (47.8 cm) and 6.5 pound (6.4 pound); 25th infant: 49.3 cm (49.0 cm) and 6.15 pound (6.15 pound); 50th infant: 50.6 cm (50.2 cm) and 7.8 pound (7.7 pound); 75th infant: 52.0 cm (51.0 cm) and 8.5 pound (8.2 pound) and 90th infant: 53.3 cm (51.9 cm) and 9.1 pound (8.10 pound), respectively.

In full-term birth, it enhanced along with the increase of the percentile standard (percentile value) of body height and body weight. As a result, in the late pregnancy, there was a significant relationship between body height and body weight.

Fourth, the total protein (g) ingested by pregnant women from daily meals during the period of the 4th to 9th months of pregnancy, and number of infants against the percentile length of birth (period from *0 to 10th Group* to *90th and over Group*) in 6 Groups were protein: 48 g; number of infant: 33 for *0 to 10th Group*; protein: 52 g; number of infant: 28 for *10th to 25th Group*; protein: 57 g; number of infant: 39 for *25th to 50th Group*; protein: 67 g; number of infant: 49 for *50th to 75th Group*; protein: 79 g; number of infant: 31 for *75th to 90th Group*; and protein: 88 g; number of infant: 14 for *90th and over Group*, respectively.

From the results of research on protein intake of pregnant women during these pregnancies, protein intake evaluated as *Good* is 70-84 g, which is too extensive. Therefore, the lower limit of protein intake assessed as *Good* will be approximately 75 g.

However, heredity is usually considered as one of the main determinants of height. Therefore, it is also necessary to consider the body height of these infants' parents. Indeed, only 138 of these 194 infants are known for the height of their parents.

Then, using these data above, there is a correlation coefficient of +0.28±0.08 between the height of the father and the height of the infant, and likewise a correlation coefficient of +0.27±0.08 between the maternal height and the infant's birth height existed. Actually, 194 out of 216 infants were within the range of percentile at birth height.

Fifth, the relationship between the body height of the mother and the average intake of total protein (g) in the prenatal meal with respect to the body height at the birth of the infant was examined.

The results were *Under 55 g protein Group (L)* (average total daily protein: under 55 g): mother's body height (tall (5 feet, 5 inches and over) 18 persons, average (5 feet, 2 inches to 5 feet, 4 inches) 17 persons, short (5 feet, 1 inch and under) 25 persons), and number of cases: 69 persons); *55 g to 74 g protein Group (M)* (average total daily protein: 55 g to 74 g): mother's body height (tall (5 feet, 5 inches and over) 47 persons, average (5 feet, 2 inches to 5 feet, 4 inches) 53 persons, short (5 feet, 1 inch and under) 50 persons), and number of cases: 80); and *75 g or more protein Group (H)* (average total daily protein: 75 g or more): mother's body height (tall (5 feet, 5 inches and over) 87 persons, average (5 feet, 2 inches to 5 feet, 4 inches) 80 persons, short (5 feet, 1 inch and under) 73 persons) and number of cases: 45), respectively.

It is clear that the amount of protein ingested from daily diets by a mother during pregnancy has a greater influence on the body height of the infant when compared to the body height of the mother.

The decrease in body height in *Group H* was proportional to the apparent decrease in protein ingestion. On the other hand, in *medium and low protein Groups* like the two *Group L* and *Group M*, the body height of the infant seems to decrease as the mother's body height increases.

From a practical nutrition standpoint, abundant protein intake during pregnancy tends to give birth to tall infants. On the contrary, it suggests that protein intake shortage has the possibility of giving birth to infant who is relatively short in spite of tall mothers.

The correlation between body length of infant and total protein is +0.80±0.03. Moreover, after removing the mother's body height, the partial correlation between body length of infant and amount of total protein in the mother's diet in the latter trimesters of pregnancy is almost the same value (+0.78±0.03).

Here, the striking relationship existed between the birth body height of the infant and the total protein intake during fetal diet. If so, the question arises as to why the protein from source which the mother ingested from the diet affects this effect more when compared to the proteins from other sources. Therefore, each protein source (g) was separated into two of protein source (g) of animal origin such as milk, cheese, meat, and domestic fowl, and protein source (g) from non-animal source. Two protein source quantities (g) of milk and cheese, respectively, were obtained separately. Similarly, all animal protein sources such as meat, fish, egg etc. were obtained by subtracting amount of grams (g) of milk and cheese from all total animal protein source (g). The correlation coefficient between these protein source groups (g) and their infant birth weight at each birth was calculated as follows: The correlation coefficient was calculated from 198 cases. Correlation coefficients (CC) between infant body length at birth and protein in meals during pregnancy were total protein: correlation coefficient (CC) +0.80, standard error (SE) ±0.03; animal protein: CC +0.68, SE ±0.04; animal protein (milk and cheese excluded): CC +0.69, SE ±0.04; milk protein: CC +0.32, SE ±0.06; nonanimal protein: CC +0.50, SE ±0.05; milk + nonanimal protein: CC +0.55, SE ±0.05; and animal protein (milk and cheese excluded) + nonanimal protein: CC +0.76, SE ±0.03, respectively.

The sixth percentile of infant body height at birth, and protein intake (g) in daily eating during pregnancy were examined. As a result, the average protein intake (g) was as follows: Percentile of body height range after birth (PHB) and average daily protein intake (g) in pregnancy was total protein (48 g), animal protein (36 g), animal protein (milk and cheese) (18 g), milk protein (20 g), nonanimal protein (13 g), milk and nonanimal protein (33 g), animal protein (milk and cheese) + nonanimal protein) (30 g) *for below PHB 10*; total protein (52 g), animal protein (37 g), animal protein (milk and cheese) (19 g), milk protein (19 g), nonanimal protein (16 g), milk and nonanimal protein (33 g), animal protein (milk and cheese) + nonanimal protein) (34 g) *for PHB 10th-25th*; total protein (57 g), animal protein (41 g), animal protein (milk and cheese) (21 g), milk protein (21 g), nonanimal protein (16 g), milk and nonanimal protein (36 g), animal protein (milk and cheese) + nonanimal protein) (37 g) *for PHB 25th-50th*; total protein (67 g), animal protein (50 g), animal protein (milk and cheese) (27 g), milk protein (23 g), nonanimal protein (18 g), milk and nonanimal protein (41 g), animal protein (milk and cheese) + nonanimal protein) (44 g) *for PHB 50th-75th*; total protein (79 g), animal protein (58 g), animal protein (milk and cheese) (35 g), milk protein (24 g), nonanimal protein (21 g), milk and nonanimal protein (45 g), animal protein (milk and cheese) + nonanimal protein) (55 g) *for PHB 75th-90th*; and total protein (88 g), animal protein (64 g), animal protein (milk and cheese) (38 g), milk protein (27 g), nonanimal protein (22 g), milk and nonanimal protein (48 g), animal protein (milk and cheese) + nonanimal protein) (59 g) *for PHB 90th or above*, respectively.

A question arises asking who can declare that "the correlation between protein in diet during pregnancy and infant body height is not caused by a few other trophic factors or factors associated with proteins in the same food, but proteins in the food are really responsible for establishing correlation."

Because, it is true that meat, eggs, milk, cheese and fish are rich in animal protein, but grains and vegetables are rich in many other functional ingredients such as anthocyanins, carotenes, vitamins, dietary fiber and minerals. The correlation coefficient of milk protein was relatively low. So, if two functional ingredients such as calcium and riboflavin (vitamin B2. **1**) (Figure 1) abundantly contained in milk are involved in the correlation coefficient, calcium and riboflavin (vitamin B2. **1**) are unlikely to be the main regulators involved in this correlation coefficient. Since each ounce(around 28.4 g) milk supplies 1 g of protein, the correlation coefficient on body height at birth will be approximately +0.32-±0.06. The total amount of protein in the fetal diet is considered to be more important factor in determining the body height at birth of an infant when compared with the intake of calcium and riboflavin (vitamin B2. **1**) in fetal stage.

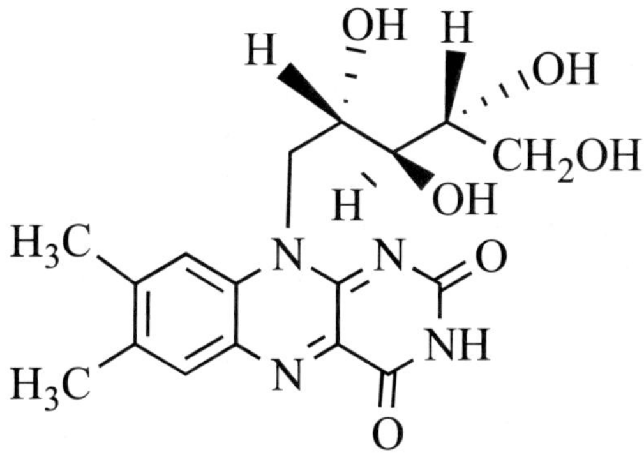

riboflavin (vitamin B2. **1**)

Figure 1. Riboflavin (vitamin B2. **1**) in animal protein.

Protein-rich foods are rich in phosphorous. Moreover, the two components of these protein and phosphorus are very closely related to food, making it difficult to identify the influence of phosphorus in such dietary study. The animal protein intake from meat and egg etc. is lower when compared to the amount of phosphorus intake in relation to various animal proteins normally taken in women's meal was investigated. If the correlation coefficient between the body height at birth and milk protein is lower compared to the correlation coefficient between birth body height and animal protein (excluding milk protein), the effect of the correlation coefficient might be resulted by the effect from the amino acid type in the animal protein rather than phosphorus in meal. Therefore, if phosphorus is the source of the correlation coefficient effect, the correlation coefficient between birth body height and milk protein might be conversely higher when compared to the correlation coefficient between birth body height and animal protein (excluding milk protein).

In addition, protein intake is more important than average caloric intake in terms of correlation between protein intake or average daily caloric intake, and body height at birth.

As far as thiamine (vitamin B1. **2**) (Figure 2) content of fetal diet, it is more difficult to obtain accurate thiamine (vitamin B1. **2**) intake from fetal history of food. Therefore, the estimated thiamine (vitamin B1. **2**) intake may be less reliable. However, according to their data, the correlation coefficient between thiamine (vitamin B1. **2**) content of the fetal diet and the body height at the birth of the infant was +0.39±0.06. Here, if the estimated value of thiamine (vitamin B1. **2**) is incorrect, distribution curves also indicate that distribution curves do not overestimate the content of thiamine (vitamin B1. **2**) in these pregnant women's diet, but are underestimating.

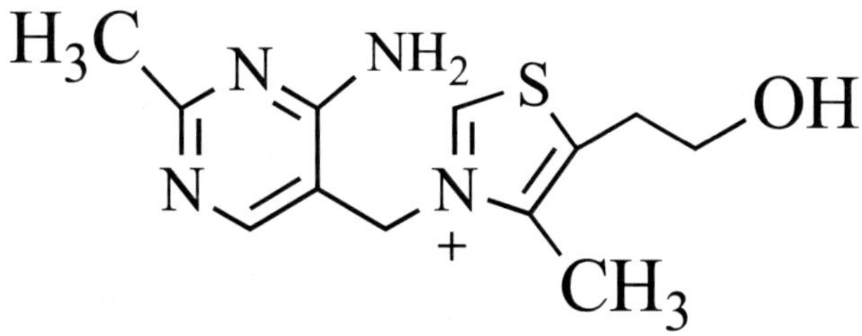

thiamine (vitamin B1. **2**)

Figure 2. Thiamine (vitamin B1. **2**) in animal protein.

Niacin (vitamin B3. nicotinic acid. **3**) (Figure 3) is present in most parts of the meat protein as a whole, so it can be one of the factors of body height at infant birth. This time, niacin (vitamin B3. nicotinic acid. **3**) content in these diets was not calculated.

However, by today, from the point of view on simple daily foods, so far it has generally been believed that proteins are not the main factor of body height at the time of infant birth. Therefore, in order to explore the main factors of body height at birth of infants, it is necessary to thoroughly reexamine whether or not dietary intake of abundant protein foods is sufficiently supplied during the fetal period.

Then, the correlation between the average protein intake (g) in the diet of pregnant women during the latter pregnancy and the birth body weight of the infant was examined. In this distribution, birth body weight gain was proportional to every 10 g increase in intake protein during fetal diet. Regarding the amount of protein arbitrarily given to the fetus from the pregnant woman's diet during gestation, protein intake of male infants was somewhat higher when compared to that (protein intake) of female infants. Birth-average weight gain was also seen with increasing 10 g of protein in the fetal diet.

It is known that the height and weight of the infant born with abundant supply of protein from the mother's diet during the fetal period are greater when compared to that (height and weight) of inadequate protein fed birth infants. However, the question comes whether the body height and weight gain of these infants is really directly linked to the health condition of the infants. It is also known that if the mother's eating habits include abundant high-quality protein, there is a good correlation between body height and body weight gain at birth, and physical development of the infant, from pediatric evaluation at birth. Namely, there is one significant correlation between both height and weight gain at birth, and the amount of protein in the daily diet of pregnant women during pregnancy. Therefore, it will be obvious that infants with a high stature and a heavy weight maintain a better health condition when compared to their infants with lower height and lighter weight.

For example, as an extreme case of a group, the average birth weight of *excellent infants* (average total protein intake of 4 months - 9 months pregnancy: 85 g/day) without any physical problems at birth or within 2 weeks of birth was 8 pounds, 2 ounces (range: 6 pounds, 10 ounces to 11 pounds, 7 ounces), and their average birth length was 50.8 cm. (range, 47.0 cm to 53.3 cm).

On the other hand, the *most deficient infants* (average total protein intake of 4 months - 9 months pregnancy: 45 g/day or less), stillborn infants who died within 2, 3 hours of birth, or on the day of birth, have a marked congenital malformation, premature birth (less than 5 pounds at birth), or functional immature. And the birth weight of the *most deficient infants* was 5 pounds, 15 ounces (range: 3 pounds, 4 ounces - 8 pounds, 15 ounces). Furthermore, the average birth height of the *most deficient infants* was 47.2 cm (range: 40.6 cm - 52.1 cm).

Regarding the entire group of 216 infants, excluding infants less than 5 pounds at birth, the relationship of birth lengths and birth weights to pediatric ratings assigned to infants at birth and within the first two weeks of life was examined.

As a result, for 5 groups of 216 infants except for infants less than 5 pounds at birth, the correlation between birth body height and birth body weight based on the four pediatric assessments assigned to infants at birth and within 2 weeks of age was 7.10 pounds (boys), 7.8 pounds (girls) and 50.6 cm (boys), 50.1 cm (girls) for *normal infants*; 8.6 pounds (boys), 7.15 pounds (girls): 51.5 cm (boys), 50.8 cm (girls) for *excellent infant*; 8.0 pounds (boys), 7.12 pounds (girls) and 51.1 cm (boys), 50.2 cm (girls) for *good infants*; 7.4 pounds (boys), 7.1 pounds (girls) and 49.9 (boys), 49.2 (girls) for *fair infants*; and 6.11 pounds (boys), 6.15 pounds (girls) and 49.1 cm (boys), 49.4 cm (girls) for the *most deficient infants*, respectively.

As a conclusion from the above results, *first*, in grouping from 216 pregnancy meals, the pregnant women who ingested the (85 g) amount, the protein recommended by the Food and Nutrition Committee of the National Research Council (NRC) during pregnancy (especially during the period from 4 to 9 months pregnancy), was only 10%. 68% of pregnant women in whole pregnancy meals during pregnancy period had protein intake less than 70 g daily and 38% of pregnant women had protein intake less than 55 g.

Second, there was a significant correlation between the protein intake in the diet of pregnant women and the birth body height of the infant. The increase in height at the time of infant birth was not directly related to the body height of the mother, but was significantly proportional to an increase in protein intake in meals during prenatal meal.

Third, regarding the relationship between the average grams of protein intake in the diet of pregnant women and the birth body weight of the infant, weight gain at infant birth was also unequivocal to the increase in protein in prenatal diet.

Fourth, protein intake during prenatal diet will be one of determinants of body length and body weight at birth. Because both body length and body weight are related to the physical evaluation of infants, protein intake in pregnant women's diet is one of the very important factors for judging the general physical condition of infants at birth.

Fifth, from this study, pregnant women meals should contain sufficient protein, from the viewpoint of the body height at birth, the body weight at birth, and the general physical health situation at birth.

From this research result, pregnant women with protein intake less than 75 g in daily life will be more likely to bring birth to infants with short stature and light weight. Therefore, for normal babies' birth, it is necessary to increase protein intake e on a daily basis during pregnancy. In addition, pregnant women will also need to receive pediatric treatment based on four pediatric evaluations [17].

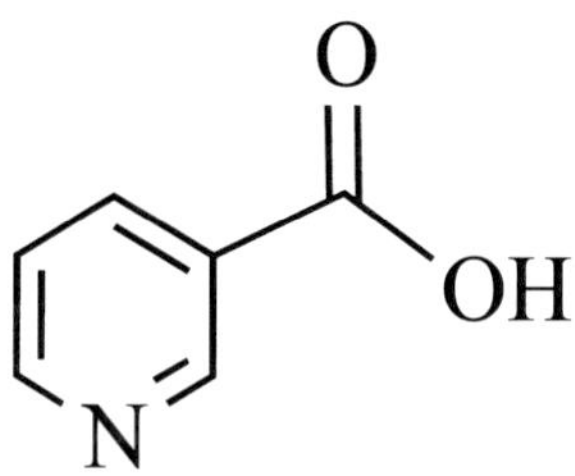

niacin (vitamin B3.
nicotinic acid. 3)

Figure 3. Niacin (vitamin B3. Nicotinic acid. **3**).

2.3.2.1. Background on Hunger

Before the survey, let's look at two backgrounds so far on hunger as follows:

2.3.2.1.1. Timing and Fetal Nutrition History

The first background is timing and the history of prenatal nutrition research.

In the late 1800s, Dr. Budan of France and Dr. Ballantine of the UK strongly proposed that fetal nutrition (maternal nutrition) is especially important for most people in the poor to be healthy pregnant women and to have a healthy early childhood. Unfortunately, however, this interest became diminished as animal experimenters could not find important developmental effects.

In the interwar period of the United States of America during the war period October 24, 1929 (later referred to as "dark Thursday"), stocks plummeted in the New York Stock Exchange of Wall Street, New York. And this economic depression (panic) spread all over the world throughout 1933, this depression continued until about 1936. This is called "the Great Depression." As a result, despite the development of industrial capitalist economy, hunger has bothered the people of the poor in Western countries to about the same extent as before the Industrial Revolution. Food or vitamin supplementation is known to be beneficial to pregnancy [15, 17, 22, 23].

Food or vitamin supplementation for pregnancy showed apparent effectiveness in World War II [24]. Specifically, in the surrounded UK, food was evenly distributed to all people not only did maternal and child health continue but also improved. On the contrary, symptoms of acute deficiency due to food deficiency showed marked deterioration. Specifically, in 18 months of Russia Leningrad siege battle [25], Dutch famine in 6 months [26, 27], and the acute food shortage in Wuppertal in Germany during the post - war chaos of 1945, the impact of hunger on baby size at birth appeared markedly [28]. Therefore, it was thought that food intake during pregnancy is involved in a large amount of infant at birth.

In addition, the discovery in the late 1950s further strengthened speculation of the effects of starvation on baby size at birth.

Although the supplement test result of protein and vitamin was good, it was not decisive [29]. Nevertheless, despite this result, new researchers who are not caught up to the previous ideas have shown the following two major studies which were not understood before [30, 31, 32, 33]. However, none of these studies also show a convincing effect of pregnancy nutrition on neonatal size. These theories mean that the fetus is a *perfect parasite* to the mother's body, and the fetus pre-empts the maternal food (feeder) as a meat and fertilizes fetal weight.

Fortunately, prenatal nutrition in pregnant women also affects a lot during the period by the peak of brain development in early childhood (the period from the first year of birth to the age after childhood to 6 years of age). Therefore, the importance of prenatal nutrition has come to be noticed again by *critical period hypothesis* in infant brain development (also called the *susceptible phase*, which is the time to decide acquisition and maturation of functions of the brain of an infant) [34]. The *critical period hypothesis* emphasizes that the specific developmental stage of the fetus is particularly important for the development of the fetus. Conversely, if the *critical period hypothesis* fails to function well in the fetal period, the fetal damage becomes unrecoverable and the subsequent developmental processes of both fetus and infant are irreversible.

Nutritional deficiency in the prenatal (embryonic) period caused damage to the placenta and made it difficult to deliver [35, 36].

In addition, each of these comparisons such as height growth between children of British from birth to 24 years old and children of Bundi, Rajasthan State, India [37], the growth rate of height between British men and women and Bundee men and women aged 1 to 25, the rate of increase in weight between British male and female children from 1 to 25 years old and Bundee male and female children, the growth curve of two sows (in the animal's belly child, the body weight of a poorly growing small sow pig (runt) is 450 g at birth and 1500 g litter breasted piglet of normal size littermate), at birth and 16 weeks thereafter, the average weight of 12 male guinea pigs born from well-nourished female parents and the average weight of the other 12 male guinea pigs born from malnourished female parents, etc. showed clearly the difference between satisfactory nutrition and nutritional deficiency in the prenatal period (embryonic period). From these experimental results, this *critical period hypothesis* has become strongly supported.

In the late 1960's, the *critical period hypothesis* was found to be involved in several cell areas as well. Initial nutrition is involved in brain development and myelination [38]; Cellular effects due to malnutrition are involved in rat development stage during malnutrition. Because early malnutrition prevented cell division and rats could not recover cell division. Furthermore, malnutrition at the late stage of growth revealed a decrease in cell size that rats cannot recover [39].

In 1968, a group of Department of Medical Microbiology and Immunology, University of California School of Medicine, LAX, USA examined the effect of maternal malnutrition before and during gestation of pregnant female albino rats, on the amount of brain DNA (brain cell number) in newborn albino rats. As a result, the effect of restriction of maternal dietary protein on weight and content of brain of newborns for 3 Diets (A, B, C) was as follows. Meal A (full pelleted diet) was offspring weights (g): 5.7 g (body) and 0.159 g (brain), and brain content of offspring: 544 μg (DNA μg) and mg (protein), respectively. Diet B (full diet, containing 27 percent protein) was offspring weights (g): 6.38 g (body) and 0.181 g (brain), and brain content of offspring: 546 μg (DNA μg) and 9.29 mg (protein), respectively. Diet C (restricted, containing 8 percent protein) was offspring weights (g): 4.46 g (body) and 0.139 g (brain), and brain content of offspring: 491 μg (DNA μg) and 7.45 mg (protein), respectively.

From the above results, first, rats given two different full meals (diet A and diet B) showed a difference in body weight and brain weight. However, the total amount of DNA, *i.e.*, the total number of brain cells, was the same. Therefore, the increased number of brain cells means a more constant index. Therefore, brain weight cannot be used as a measure of the number of brain cells.

Second, regarding meal B (full diet with 27% protein) and meal C (restricted diet containing 8% protein), the weight loss of newborns is proportional to the same decrease in total protein content. The change in weight loss of all these newborns is statistically significant.

The amount of DNA (DNA 491 μg) in the brain of meal C (diet restricted diet containing 8% protein) having restricted diet decreased also remarkably 10% when compared to the amount of brain DNA (DNA 546 μg) in meal B (full diet containing 27% protein). However, the difference in the amount of DNA in the brain between meal C (restricted diet containing 8% protein) and meal B (full diet containing 27% protein) is not evident. Therefore, it means that the amount of DNA in the brain cannot be used as a measure of brain weight.

Neonatal brain cells at birth are known to be mainly neurons [40]. Therefore, DNA reduction in the brain may actually affect the number of neurons. Furthermore, the number of neurons in the brain after birth essentially does not increase by dividing the number of neurons in the brain more than after birth. Therefore, neuron deficiency at birth will last throughout the life of the albino rats.

Maternal brain neuron deficiency may contribute to behavioral disturbances from previously known protein deficiency mothers to offspring.

Changes in protein mass from meal C (restricted diet containing 8% protein) to meal B (full diet containing 27% protein) increased by 24%, whereas changes in DNA amount increased by 11%. This increase in the amount of protein and DNA indicate not only that the number of cells has changed but also that the cells are quantitatively different. It is not yet known whether quantitative changes in the amounts of these protein and DNA are irreversible or whether they merely indicate a delay in maturation. However, 3-month-old albino rats with meal C (restricted diet containing 8% protein) had a higher gait abnormality and the response to environmental stimulation when compared to 3-month old albino rats of meal B (full diet containing 27% protein) [41].

In 1966, a group from Department of Physiology, London Hospital Medical College, University of London, UK examined the late stage of brain development, that is, the collapse deposition of myelin *which is a component of the myelin sheath* by using many literatures, followed by the investigation in accordance with the hypothesis regarding the period of maximum vulnerability of myelin formation during the major brain's growth period on the influence of certain external factors.

As a result, from these studies on relative metabolic stability of myelin sheath *which is the sheath surrounding nerve fiber conveying information on the nerve* and chemical structure of myelin sheath, the myelin content of brain was suggested to decrease only during myelination period. Therefore, the importance of timing of prenatal nutrition, in particular, is the period of myelination as a vulnerable period in brain development.

However, even limitations such as small dietary restrictions received during this vulnerable period of brain development may have a sustained impact on subsequent intellectual ability. The hypothesis of physical growth of both brain and body was not systematically investigated [42].

In 1985, a research group at Gertrude H. Sergievsky Center of Columbia University, New York, USA examined the effects of early nutrition on neurological and mental performance in humans focusing on the effects of early nutrition throughout the four periods of before and after mother's conception (periconception), embryonic phase, foetal phase, and postnatal phase:

The first one is before and after mother's conception (periconception): In general, three representative diseases (iodine deficiency, insulin deficiency, and hyperphenylalaninemia) at the conception stage are associated with specific metabolic problems.

First, iodine deficiency before and after conception in mother is a congenital disease associated with hypothyroidism. It is associated with cretinism with offspring such as body malformations and idiotism [43].

Second, regarding mother's insulin deficiency resulting in insulin-dependent diabetes, it is thought that insulin-dependent diabetes, uncontrolled by the mother, affects development before pregnancy [44].

Third, phenylketonuria in a pregnant woman exposes her offspring *in utero* to hyperphenylalaninemia. In general, it is known that high blood phenylalanine levels in humans for a long period of time may inhibit brain development and cause intellectual impairment. Since many women with phenylketonuria (PKU) will have their own children, the effects of maternal phenylketonuria (PKU) and hyperphenylalaninemia on such maternal offspring, *i.e.*, their effects of outcomes on both maternal phenylketonuria (PKU) and hyperphenylalaninemia-untreated pregnancy, and maternal phenylketonuria (PKU) and hyperphenylalaninemia-treated pregnancy were investigated.

Among 524 pregnant women, the phenylketonuric disease history of pregnant women was 369 and 155 pregnant women with phenylketonuria. Of the 155 pregnant women with phenylketonuria, 34 pregnant women started the *low phenylalanine diet* just before or just after pregnancy was established.

As a result, it was shown that maternal phenylketonuria and hyperphenylalaninemia-untreated pregnant women have higher incidence of mental retardation, microcephaly and congenital heart disease when compared to those (incidences) of normal pregnant women. Increased incidences on these two types of phenylketonuria and hyper-phenylalaninemia were correlated with maternal blood phenylalanine levels. Ninety-five percent of mothers with blood phenylalanine 20 mg/dL or more had at least one child with mental retardation. The bias introduced by case detection did not explain these results.

From these results, it is unclear whether a diet started after conception would be useful. However, the treatment for two maternal phenylketonuria and hyperphenylalaninemia started before conception is essential and should be evaluated [45].

The second is the embryonic phase: At this embryonic stage, two completely different types of acute nutrient deficiency and chronic nutrient deficiency suggest a role for nutrition in the developmental form of the central nervous system (CNS).

First, maternal acute starvation affects both the length of pregnancy and fetal organogenesis. Hunger is a pathological condition caused by the lack of essential nutrients and water that are vital for human beings to survive. Thus, among pregnant women who were exposed to the *"the Dutch famine (starving in the Netherlands)"* who starved during the fetal period born in February 1945 to March 1946, during the first three months of pregnancy (trimester) exposure, pregnant women alone suffered a number of injuries, including unusually excessive extra-low birth weight premature infants, excessive stillborn infants and the first week of death after birth [46].

It is not known why these injuries develop in the first three months (first trimester). However, among the follow-up causes of death for those exposed to Dutch famine during the first trimester, exposure to excessive *Dutch famine* caused central nervous system (CNS) disorders. This is because, among the 19-year-old male survivors, excessive neural tube defects and cerebral infantile palsy (cerebral palsy. CP) have been identified [47].

Excessive obesity was identified among fetal survivors who were exposed to *Dutch famine* during the embryonic period of the pregnant woman [48]. This result is reproduced experimentally using rats exposed to *Dutch famine* [49].

Second, chronic malnutrition caused by chronic exposure to essential nutrient deficiencies in the maternal diet prior to birth is thought to be the cause of neural tube defects such as spondylosis and anencephaly. This hypothesis for chronic malnutrition has been considered correct from the perspective of social starvation, geographical bias, and temporal and chronological variation.

The mother's hyperphenylalaninemia and preconceptional iodine deficiency are the basis for all offspring to develop these two diseases. All children born to a group of untreated mothers with iodine deficiency in New Guinea have psychometric impairments when compared to children from a group of mothers who received random iodinated oil injections before pregnancy [50]. Therefore, iodine deficiency is a typical prenatal dietary disorder that directly affects both neurological function and mental function.

Third is the fetal phase: The two major causes of illness due to dietary essential nutrient deficiencies in prenatal maternal fetus are acute hunger and chronic maternal malnutrition.

The main clinical interest in the fetal phase is the relationship between poor maternal nutrition and low birth weight, followed by relationship between depression and low birth weight. Furthermore, the relationship between an increase in birth weight and improvement of the mind (depression) was investigated. It is known that the relationship between birth weight and subsequent mental behavior (mental disorder) including psychotic disorder, anxiety disorder, drug addiction *etc.* is complicated.

Therefore, several casual routes need to be considered that are listed below:

First, a common cause - chromosomal abnormalities or intrauterine lesions - cause both low birth weight and mental retardation (intellectual disorder). Thus, in some forms of mental retardation associated with low birth weight, chromosomal abnormalities are prodromal symptoms that are manifested as an antecedent of the both intrauterine growth retardation and mental retardation.

This chromosomal aberration or intrauterine lesion model did not show a significant correlation between prenatal maternal as well as fetal nutrition, intrauterine growth retardation and the onset of mental retardation. However, this relationship is excellent in the interpretation of the association between prenatal pregnant women and the fetus (in humans, about 3 months after conception), and intrauterine fetal dysfunction and intellectual developmental disorder (mental retardation). If these observations are not considered then, the true causality will be mistakenly more difficult to assess.

Second, some other factors likely to be associated with malnutrition cause significant premature infants, and very low birth weight. Extremely low birth weight infant less than 1500 g will undoubtedly increase the risk of mental retardation and cerebral palsy. It may be that preterm birth (prematurity), immaturity and vulnerability are likely to be susceptible to these etiologies of the risk for both mental retardation and cerebral palsy. In the early 1980's, among very low birth weight infants, mental retardation incidence accounted for approximately 1% of the births of very low birth weight in New York City. However, in the 1960s, the risk of severe mental retardation among very low birth weight infants was as high as about 4-5%. These very low birth weight infants almost always had severe anoxia and associated neuropathy. In contrast, in the general birth population, the risk of mental retardation was less than 0.05%.

As for very low birth weight infants and the risk of severe mental retardation, the relationship between the incidence of preterm (premature) low birth weight infants and the maternal diet may be weak. This is because pregnant women who were exposed to *Dutch famine* during the prenatal period only shortened on average 4 days gestation. Among chronic malnourished pregnant women, supplementation with nutritional supplements during pregnancy hardly increased the mean duration of pregnancy.

In Japan after World War II (WWII) in 1945, it is important to ascertain whether the increase in average birth weight after improved economic and health status by diet modification is due to prolongation of pregnancy or better fetal development. According to birth weight records on pregnancy period for 20 years of pregnancy at three major obstetric hospitals in Japan, not only did recovery from the supply shortage during WWII occurred, but it also increased the average birth weight beyond pre-war levels. The pregnancy period was not extended. However, the growth curve of pregnancy showed a marked increase in weight during the pregnancy period in the second half of the third trimester (late gestation period. 29 weeks onwards) which revealed that the socioeconomic factors have a great influence on fetal growth. Here are the following hypotheses about fetal development: That is, "the difference in average birth weight of the population is due to difference in time when growth starts to fall below the optimal level at the end of late pregnancy period." Japan's average birth weight gain after World War II is in good agreement with this hypothesis which is due to socioeconomic factors. In addition, with regard to six-year-old children born at the same time during the pregnancy period during the second half of the third trimester, at the follow-up after six years, even at the age of six, the height and weight gain of children (newborn infants at that time) who showed a marked increase in weight are higher when compared to those (newborn infants at that time) who did not show weight gain during the same period of pregnancy [51].

Third, there is a direct correlation between depressed mental performance (mental behavior loss) and/or mild mental retardation, and depressed birthweight (birth weight loss). In this hypothesis, there is a partial relationship between low birthweight and mild mental retardation, poverty and poor dietary circumstances (poor eating environment). The third model is a malnutrition model on fetal growth retardation (fetal growth delay) that leads to irreversible depletion of brain cell numbers including the fetal brain, and subsequently induction to a postnatal mental deterioration [52].

The fourth is the postnatal phase: It is very difficult to distinguish whether mental retardation is due to the effects of prenatal or postnatal diet. From experimental biochemical studies of brain cell components, the malnutrition during the prenatal critical period of rapid brain cell proliferation and the early postnatal critical period can cause irreversible damage [52].

In general, the action of dietary supplements is moderate and mainly effective for motor function, and furthermore this effect is only evident during the use of dietary supplements. On the contrary, the Einstein scale of sensorimotor intelligence, which is most closely related to cognition, gave contradictory results. Indeed, malnutrition probably reduces concurrent motivation and arousal. However, the restorative effect of dietary supplements on these concurrent motivations and awakenings may not be long-term.

According to long-term observational studies in Mexican villages, there is a relationship between nutritional and social environmental aspects, and their combined impact on mental function in the environmental aspects. Based on this fact, mental deterioration was certainly related to poor nutrition. However, mental dysfunction due to malnutrition always appeared only in the missing time of social stimuli such as *Dutch famine* [53].

In conclusion from many of the above results, specific dietary nutrient deprivation and metabolic imbalances underlie many forms of mental retardation or mental deterioration. Currently, as far as these are understood, these nutrient deprivation and metabolic imbalances are associated with the very early stages of pregnancy, such as periconceptional phase or the phase of embryogenesis. In these mentally retarded and impaired mental disorders, the basis of prevention, such as essential nutrient supplementation, is far more effective than treatment. Apart from these effects during early pregnancy, acute or chronic malnutrition at prenatal, fetal and early postnatal stages has been shown to be a permanent cause of mental decline. However, when chronic malnutrition is combined with social deficits, childhood cognitive ability may decline even after adulthood [16, 23, 54].

2.3.2.1.2. The Relationship between Fetal Developmental Stages and the Effects of Fetal Nutrition under the Disastrous Situation of the Dutch Famine Winter of 1944-1945

As mentioned above, *Dutch famine* from 1944 to 1945 increased low birth weight infants. And one of the main causes of this was exposure during the third trimester of pregnancy [27].

In 1994, a group of Gertrude H. Sergievsky Center of Columbia University Medical Center, USA examined relationship between developmental stage of fetus and influence of intrathecal nutrition in tragic circumstances of the Dutch Hunger Winter of 1944-1945. The research group investigated some of their clinical histories, not for its own sake, but to reveal the relationship between a starvation period and episode of epidemiological specific disease. Therefore, the main objective of this study is to clarify the correlation between the timing of development including duration, severity, and type under nutritional hunger, and the influence of fetal nutrition (maternal nutrition) [23].

As a result, the main symptoms that are likely to develop during the three stages of pregnancy due to starvation are:

First, periconceptional (pre- and post-pregnancy) are fertility, organic encephalopathy (organic brain disorder. WHO (World Health Organization) defined mainly 18 kinds of tropical diseases that must be controlled such as Dengue fever, lymphatic filariasis, Chagas disease, *etc.*) – *i.e.*, *neglected tropical diseases* (*NTDs*) -, schizophrenia, schizophrenic personality disorder, and antisocial personality disorder.

Second, first trimester pregnancy (pregnancy for the first 3 months) is the length of pregnancy (premature birth), stillbirth, first week mortality increase due to infectious disease, and increased obesity.

Third, third trimester pregnancy is maternal weight gain, birth increased weight including second generation, mortality increase at 0-3 months after birth, and decreased obesity [23].

The above epidemiological analysis lacks the second trimester pregnancy. This may be because the symptoms of famine exposure in the first trimester pregnancy may be transferred to the second trimester pregnancy. However, their epidemiological validation has again shown a relationship between fetal developmental stages and the effects of prenatal nutrition. Collectively, from an epidemiological point of view, it shows how the effects of prenatal nutrition are important for the developmental stage of the fetus [23].

2.3.2.2. Effects of Prenatal (Fetal) Diet on Mother and Child

To date, the relationship of fetal stage (prenatal) process, outcome of pregnant mother and fetus with nutrition has been discussed much. However, the conclusion of these relationships is contradictory.

First, in 1941 and 1943, separately, it was confirmed that there was a significant relationship between the pregnant mother's diet and the mother's complications and incidence of fetal abnormality. In 1941, a group of Departments of Paediatrics and Obstetrics, University of Toronto, Canada conducted an epidemiological study on the prenatal diet of 400 low-income women in order to know the effect of prenatal diet on mothers and babies. The first group taking a meager meal was treated as a *Control Group*. The mother (*Group 2*) taking a meager meal with supplemental diet was improved during the last 3 or 4 months of pregnancy while the *Group 3*, who is doing a moderately good prenatal diet, was improved only by education.

Throughout the course of pregnancy, mothers who used diet by supplements (*Group 2*) or mothers who had a good diet (*Group 3*) maintained better health than *Group 1* health, and had few complications. *Group 2* and *Group 3* had lower obstetric risk when compared to that (obstetric risk) of *Group*. The incidence of miscarriage, stillbirth and preterm birth was significantly lower in mothers who had dietary supplements (*Group 2*) or mothers with good diet (*Group 3*) than *Group 1*. In addition, the incidence of illness in infants up to 6 months of age and the number of deaths from these diseases in *Group 1* were markedly higher than *Group 2* and *Group 3*.

Based on the above results, it was suggested that a good diet during pregnancy reduces incidence of miscarriage, stillbirth, preterm birth and obstetric risk, *etc.*, and is indispensable for maintaining the health of mothers and fetuses [55].

2.3.2.3. Fetal Disorder Due to Prenatal Nutritional Deficiency of Pregnant Womens

Fetal growth depends on good diet in a much broader range than maintenance. At the early stage of pregnancy, the fertilized eggs contains some nutrients in themselves, however, in later stages the eggs must rely on the nutrients from mother to grow and develop fully.

It has been widely thought that the degree of fetal dependence (effect) on the relationship between the mother and the fetus and the mother's meal depends on the growth of the fetus, the fetal disease, the mortality rate of the fetus, the health condition of the newborn after birth and the development of neonatal organs including the brain. Hence, it is important to understand the interrelationship between mother & fetus or neonate, including the extent of fetus's dependence (influence) on mother's diet, before understanding the role of nutrition during pregnancy.

The degree of fetal dependence (effect) on the interaction between mother and fetua, as well as on mother's diet must be determined through observation of prenatal diet and general health. Both these prenatal diets and general health observations may be tightly regulated by the mothers' prejudiced situation (to solitary enemies).

Therefore, a satisfying study of the effects of nutrition on fetal growth and development, from a third party perspective, must conduct an epidemiological investigation according to the following three situations: (1) Influence of health condition and nutrition of the mother before pregnancy and pregnancy on the prenatal course of the newborn and the development of the fetus. (2) Nutritional requirement for pregnancy and relationship between pregnancy nutritional status and pregnancy requirement of mother. (3) Relative importance of essential nutrients that must be ingested from food to preserve pregnancy, parturition, labor, puerperal processes and fetal development and infant health, *i.e.*, growth and body maintenance.

To date, there are many papers on infant development and health concerning prenatal nutrition related to the fetus. However, very few papers on fetal disorders due to prenatal nutritional deficiency are known.

Regarding fetal disorders due to prenatal nutritional deficiencies, the research group at the University of Wisconsin Agricultural Experiment Station examined the effects of different feed distribution on growth and breeding [56]. As a result, it was discovered that young cows (heifers) raised in maize without premature births produce healthy calves of normal size at the expiration of pregnancy, and that calves can stomach within 1 hour after birth to suck on breast milk. Nevertheless, both mother cattle and calves lived normally with full development. On the other hand, young cows (heifers) without birth experience raised in wheat produced premature birth, or the calf born was small, and the probability of death within several hours after birth was high. Young cows fed with oat plant feed or a mixture of three cereals gave birth to weak calves or still births.

The experiment was continued, and the cows were administered different feed distributions. In the following year, these cows repeated the same symptoms as the previous reproductive records of cows.

Likewise, inappropriate nutrition of pregnant women during prenatal period is known to damage in similar way to human fetuses [57], human foetal rickets [58] and damage in foetal life [59].

In addition, nutritional requirements of pregnant women were also confirmed from metabolic studies on pregnant women [18, 60].

The pregnant mother's diet was involved in a lot of maternal health status during pregnancy, newborn's birth status and infant's condition during months of life [55].

2.3.2.4. Oral Administration of Nutritional Supplements and Toxemia of Pregnancy

In 1942, a group of The People’s League of Health, UK examined the relationship between oral administration of supplement and incidence of toxemia in pregnancy based on hypertension diagnostic treatment methods.

The interim report from the Committee of Health People's Federation of UK showed an interesting statistical data on the effect of improving prenatal diet by using supplements as follows [61]:

It is questionable if the committee really helps pregnancy, labor, and newborns by adding supplements such as vitamins and minerals to the diet. Subsequently, committee decided the prescription dose of vitamins and minerals needed to ascertain these questions. The prescription dose of daily supplements used for the experiment was as follows:

Saccharified iron carbonate 8 g (iron: 1.2 g) is equivalent to 0.26 g ferrous iron.

Calcium lactate 30 g (calcium: 2 g) is equivalent to 0.26 g calcium.

Trace amounts of iodine, manganese, copper.

Vitamin B1 adsorbate containing all the vitamin B1 complex factors (standardized with vitamin B1 amount 200 IU/g) 15 g is equivalent to 1 g of vitamin B1.

Ascorbic acid (vitamin C. **4**) (Figure 4) is administered 100 mg.

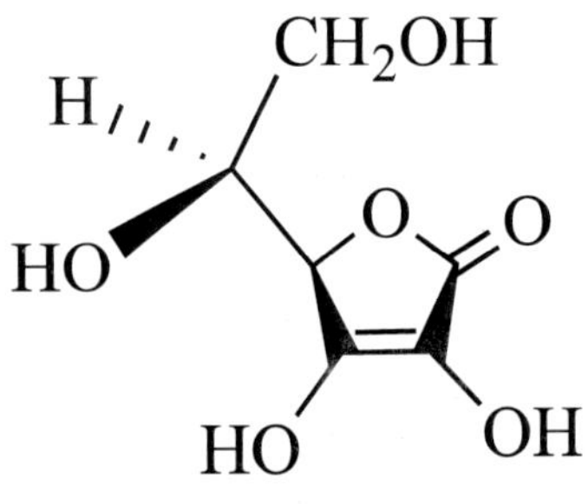

ascorbic acid (vitamin C. 4)

Figure 4. Ascorbic acid (vitamin C. **4**).

6 g of halibut oil (vitamin A: 52,000 IU/g; vitamin D: 2,500 IU/g) is equivalent to vitamin A + vitamin D 0.36 g.

Incidentally, each hospital classified pregnant women registered in the clinic before birth alternately into separate lists and classified them into two main groups. *Group 1* pregnant women did not receive supplements as *controls*. *Group 2* pregnant women took supplements with meals. *Group 1* and *group 2* were subdivided into first pregnant women (primigravidae) and multiparae, respectively. In addition, *Group 1* and *Group 2* have been subdivided into 3 sections under 25 years old, 25 years old to 30 years old, and over 30 years old, respectively. All pregnant women who are not in good health or pregnant women who are expected to give birth within 16 weeks have been excluded from the experiment.

2.3.2.4.1. Toxemia of Pregnancy

The symptoms of toxemia of pregnancy (preeclampsia) comprises two symptoms: 1. a pregnant woman who showed albuminuria (albumin urine which is mainly used as a measurement for early detection of diabetic nephropathy), hypertension with or without edema (systolic blood pressure above 140 mm Hg or 90 mm Hg diastolic blood pressure). 2. a pregnant woman who does not have high blood pressure, but diagnosis was based on albuminuria.

First, in 1530 primary pregnant women who received nutritional supplements, the toxemia rate was 27.1%. On the other hand, among the 1512 first pregnant women who did not receive supplementary diet, the proportion of toxemia rate was 31.7%, the standard deviation (S.D.) was 4.6 ±1.7%.

Regarding the main reason for the standard deviation (S.D.) (4.6 ± 1.7%) in toxemia between both primigravidae, most pregnant women aged 25 to 30 years old used nutritional supplements. In fact, the standard deviation (S.D.) in toxemia between pregnant women between the ages of 25 and 30 showed a very large difference (7.7 ± 2.6%).

However, multiparae, there was no difference in toxemia rate between the two groups, *nutritional supplements taking Group* and *non-nutritional supplements taking Group*. In both groups of 980 *nutritional supplements taking Group* and 999 *non-nutritional supplements taking Group*, the incidence of toxemia was both 21.8%.

Second, recently, it is found that diagnosis of toxemia cannot be judged on measuring only hypertension which has been used for many years. Toxemia occurs not only in intrinsic or specific pregnancy toxemia but also in essential hypertension, which is a condition where the cause of high blood pressure is not clear. Therefore, diagnosis of toxemia cannot depend only on high blood pressure measurement.

Even if pregnant women with essential hypertension which is the only clinical abnormality are excluded from the above group, general hypertension is also caused by albuminuria, edema, *etc*.

Treatment of symptoms of hypertension due to etiology such as those mentioned above such as albuminuria and edema could exclude some cases diagnosed hypertension due to toxemia.

Such diagnostic treatment for hypertension has the advantage that diagnosis of toxemia can be easily separated from the etiology such as albuminuria and edema based on proper and safe basis.

First, regarding albuminuria with or without hypertension in both the *primips (primigravida) Group taking dietary supplement* and the *primips (primigravida) Group taking non-dietary supplement* (controls), the standard error (S.E.) of the *primigravida Group receiving dietary supplement* (5.4%) and the *primigravida Group receiving non-dietary supplement (controls)* (7.4%) was 2.0 ± 0.9. These observations suggest that the odds are close to 40 to 1 for the result obtained by mere coincidence.

Second, regarding albuminuria with or without hypertension in both the *multips (parous women) Group taking dietary supplement* and the *multips (parous women) Group taking non-dietary supplement* (controls), the standard error (S.E.) of the *primigravida Group receiving dietary supplement* (3.6%) and the *primigravida Group receiving non-dietary supplement (controls)* (5.2%), but not to a significant degree, was 1.6± 0.9. Therefore, pregnant women receiving *dietary supplements* are protected from the higher risk of toxemia at a rate (proportion) of approximately 30% when compared to the risk of *non-nutritional supplement* pregnant women.

Following postpartum sepsis (puerperal sepsis), toxemia of pregnancy is the second leading cause of death, accounting for approximately 20% of maternal mortality (around a fifth of the total), in addition to the cause of death from chronic health problems after childbirth.

Third, in further classification based on criteria generally accepted for preeclampsia which is a disease characterized by high blood pressure and proteinuria during pregnancy and increases the risk of outcome failure of both the pregnant women and neonates, the incidence of hypertension, edema, and toxemia with albuminuria was as follows:

First, the first pregnant Group taking nutritional supplement group: 4.51%; the first pregnant Group taking non-nutritional supplement Group: 6.42%; standard error (S.E.): 1.91 ± 0.82.

Second, nutritional supplement (supplement) taking Group of multipara (primipara): 3.16%; non-nutritional supplement taking of multipara (primipara)(control): 4.60%; standard error (S.E.): 1.44 ± 0.87.

2.3.2.4.2. Infant

First, on premature babies: the committee found evidence that diet modification during pregnant mothers is statistically significant for the infant's normal development. It was suggested that pregnant women can reduce the birth of premature infants by diet therapy.

In fact, 308 primigravidae (standard error: 20.1 ± 1.10) out of the *first pregnant women (primigravidae) dietary supplement taking Group* (1529 primigravidae) finished birth on early 40 weeks before the expected delivery date. On the other hand, 361 *primigravidae* (standard error: 23.9 ± 1.10) out of the first pregnant women (1512 *primigravidae*) *taking non-nutritional supplements primigravidae (control)* were premature births.

The trends related to *dietary supplement taking Group* and *non-dietary supplement taking Group* of *multiparae (primiparae)* were similar to those (trends) of the first pregnant women (*primigravidae*). Namely, the standard error of the *dietary supplement taking Group* was 20.1 ± 1.33, and the *non-dietary supplement taking Group* was standard error 24.2 ± 1.33. The standard error for both the *first pregnant women (primigravidae)* and *multiparae (primiparae)* was greater fluctuation than mere chance fluctuation.

The *dietary supplement taking Group* had a relatively higher proportion of maturity birth than the *non-dietary supplement taking Group.*

This is because 50% of infant deaths in less than a month are due to infant deaths from premature infants in *non-dietary supplement taking Group*.

Second, on birth-weight of baby: For primigravidae of all ages, the difference of birth-weight of baby was slight - 7.18±0.03 lb. for the *dietary supplement taking Group*; 7.17±0.03 lb. for the *non-dietary supplement taking Group (controls)*. However, on pregnant women age 30 and over, birth-weight of baby (7.17±0.7 lb.) in the *dietary supplement taking Group* indicated a heavier range when compared to birth-weight of baby (6.99±0.07 lb.) in the *non-dietary supplement taking Group (controls)*. The difference between both is 0.18 pounds; on the contrary, this difference has an important meaning.

Like the first pregnant woman (primigravidae) of all ages, the birth weight difference between the *dietary supplement taking Group* and *non-dietary supplement taking Group (controls)* of multiparae is 0.07 ± 0.05 pounds, and the birth weight difference between both *Groups* is not significant. However, the tendency of this difference value favors the *dietary supplement taking Group* of multiparae. Indeed, in the three age groups of the four age groups of multiparae, the birth weight of the neonates in the *dietary supplement taking Group* was somewhat heavier when compared to that (birth weight of the neonates) of *non-dietary supplement taking Group (controls)*.

Incidentally, there was a considerable difference in the birth weight of newborn babies at different hospitals in the UK. For example, the average birth weight for the first pregnant women (primigravidae) in hospital B was 6.98 pounds. However, the birth weight average of newborns of the first pregnant women (primigravidae) at hospital G and hospital J were 7.22 pounds and 7.42 pounds, respectively. Furthermore, at these three hospitals (B, G, J), the birth weight average for newborn babies corresponding to the class of multiparae were 7.43 pounds, 7.62 pounds and 7.89 pounds, respectively.

The differences in birth weight average values between the first pregnant women (primigravidae) in these three different hospitals, or between multiparae, and the differences in birth weight average value between first pregnant women (primigravidae) and multiparae in corresponding hospitals are statistically significant, and its deviation deserves further investigation.

2.3.2.4.3. Adverse Effect

According to the committee, during pregnancy, it was unable to find evidence that vitamin and mineral oral administration to the pregnant women had a significant impact on the risk of side effects such as fever after birth and sepsis.

At the same time, administration of vitamins and minerals to the pregnant women did not have a big influence on the nature or working hours of pregnant women.

2.3.2.4.4. Conclusion

Collectively, the oral administration of a dietary supplement to pregnant women proposed by the committee was accompanied by a decrease in the incidence of hypertension, edema, and toxemia accompanied by albuminuria, an increase in neonatal birth weight, and a reduction in infant mortality by premature infants less than a month, *etc.* [21, 61].

2.3.2.5. Nutrition during Pregnancy and Physical Condition of Infant

In 1943, a group of Department of Child Hygiene, School of Public Health, Department of Obstetrics, School of Medicine, Harvard University, Boston, USA examined nutrition during pregnancy and physical condition of infant.

The results were as follows:

1) There was a statistically significant correlation between the mother's diet during pregnancy and the infant's physical condition at birth.
2) When pregnant mothers have poor or very poor food intake, they can not provide enough essential nutrients for the fetus. So the infant becomes immature infant. In fact, of the 216 pregnant women surveyed, all immature infants died several days after birth

except one infant. Most causes of infant death were severe congenital defects. All premature infants born to mothers who had a very inadequate diet during pregnancy and all functional premature infants were very difficult to grow.

3) When pregnant mother's diet is excellent or good, mother's infant will probably be in good or excellent physical condition.
   However, it may happen occasionally that a mother with excellent or good diet during pregnancy gives birth to a physically deconditioned baby. Because, in this epidemiological analysis, one premature infant (premature baby) out of 216 infants dies from other diseases rather than severe congenital defect (birth defects).
4) It was found that there was a statistically significant relationship between prenatal diet and the course of pregnancy. However, this relationship is different from what exists between prenatal dietary assessment and the physical condition of the infant. This indicates that the fetus suffers more than the mother if nutrition during pregnancy is inadequate.
5) In this study, mothers who were regarded as having a good or excellent diet during pregnancy did not suffer from pre-eclampsia (pregnancy toxemia). On the other hand, around 50% of infants born to a mother who ate a very poor diet from a poor diet during pregnancy had pre-eclampsia.
6) It was found that there was no statistically significant association between prenatal nutrition, and the duration and characteristics of parturition. Despite the fact that, on an average, mothers who ate a poor diet or very poor diet during pregnancy have given birth to a smaller infant than a mother whose diet was considered good or excellent,
7) There was no statistical significance between prenatal nutrition and the postpartum course. There seems to be a trend towards a relationship between prenatal nutrition and the occurrence of major complications in the postpartum period, which is the period of time until the changes in maternal genital and whole body caused by

pregnancy and labor return to the pre-pregnancy state, and usually 6 to 8 weeks [21, 31].

2.4. Arginine Paradox: Free Radicals Regulate the Aging Process

In traditional Chinese medicine (TCM) and folklore medicine, garlic (*Allium sativum*. dà suàn in Chinese) which gives off a unique strong scent has been used for prevention and treatment of a wide variety of diseases such as cold, bacteriostasis of digestive organs such as detoxified intestines and Shigella. L-Arginine (L-Arg. **5**) (Figure 5) contained in garlic is known as a semiessential amino acid and various pharmacological effects are known [62]. The role of L-arginine (L-Arg. **5**) in disease treatment is revealed below.

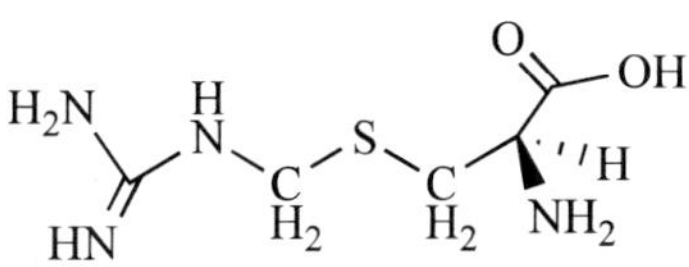

arginine (L-Arg. **5**)

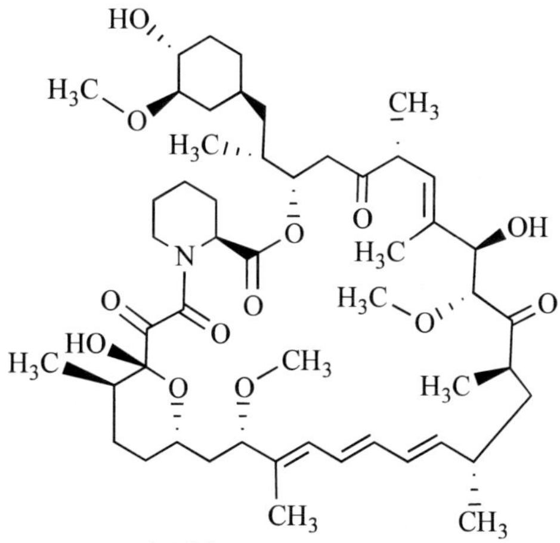

rapamycin (**6**)

Figure 5. Arginine (L-Arg. **5**) and rapamycin (**6**).

Generally, it is known that the overproduction of reactive oxygen species (ROS) leads to oxidative stress, resulting in a variety of changes in the cell conversion due to external as well as internal environmental factors. Oxidative stress thus contributes to cell injury and hence is related to chronic diseases including cancer, diabetes, Alzheimer's disease and other diseases [63]. These diseases are characterized by an imbalance between the antioxidant enzyme system and ROS production, resulting in further damage [64]. It was shown that cellular metabolites might play a major role in oxidative tissue damage [65, 66].

Natural antioxidants are known to exist in plants, animals, and also microorganisms [67, 68, 69]. L-Arginine (L-Arg. **5**) as a semiessential amino acid is readily available from diverse food sources and plays an important functional role regarding the function to adjust body condition in living organisms as well as in various diseases [70, 71, 72].

As L-arginine (L-Arg. **5**) is used as a biosynthetic precursor of secondary metabolite nitric oxide (NO) (*i.e.,* a substrate of the NO synthesis enzyme) in mammals, L-arginine (L-Arg. **5**) has been widely studied to develop the diverse bioactive compounds.

In general, it has long been thought that the chronic supply of exogenous L-arginine (L-Arg. **5**) further increases nitric oxide (NO) production, but contrary to this idea, the acute supply of exogenous L-arginine (L-Arg. **5**) rather improved nitric oxide (NO) production [73]. This phenomenon is known as arginine paradox.

The concentration of L-arginine (L-Arg. **5**) determines directly both arginase activity, and the production of nitric oxide (NO), urea of the chief solid component of mammalian urine, citrulline of an amino acid that does not occur in proteins but is an intermediate in the conversion of ornithine to arginine, and ornithine of basic amino acid belonging to the urea cycle [74].

Additionally, L-arginine (L-Arg. **5**) is involved in insulin resistance [75, 76], heat stress [77], oxidative stress [78], and other environmental stress such as residential environment, commuting environment and work environment [79].

It suggests that the reason that L-arginine (L-Arg. **5**) manifests many kinds of physiological functions as described above is that L-arginine (L-Arg. **5**) can be attributed to some aging or its regulatory effect on resistance-related genes.

Dietary L-arginine (L-Arg. **5**) could activate the pathway target of immunosuppressive agent rapamycin (**6**) (Figure 5) which is one macrolide compound produced by *Streptomyces hygroscopicus*. L-arginine (L-Arg. **5**) promote the target of rapamycin (**6**) (TOR)-related protein synthesis in a freshwater fish *Megalobrama amblycephala* [80].

L-Arginine (L-Arg. **5**) supplementation was able to alleviate liver thermal stress of Pekin duck. From the above many pharmacological actions, it is suggested that the main action mechanism of L-arginine (L-Arg. **5**) is due to NO production *in vivo*.

NO can increase longevity, enhance stress resistance or produce other beneficial consequences [81, 82, 83].

L-Arginine (L-Arg. **5**) is used for synthesis of nitric oxide (NO) by nitric oxide synthase (NOS) in diverse organisms, ranging from yeasts to mammals. However, *Caenorhabditis elegans* cannot synthesize nitric oxide (NO), because *C. elegans* lacks nitric oxide synthase (NOS) [84].

Here, one question that says "*C. elegans* can increase environmental stress tolerance by using L-arginine (L-Arg. **4**) directly, even if nitric oxide (NO) does not exist?" will come out.

To test this hypothesis, the *C. elegans* were fed with live OP50 *Escherichia coli* as neither *C. elegans* nor *Escherichia coli* can produce nitric oxide (NO).

These *C. elegans* lived longer and enhanced activity of reactive oxygen species (ROS) detoxification enzymes, and a lower production of reactive oxygen species (ROS).

As several factors caused longevity or increased stress resistance, some aging-associated genes or antioxidant genes were upregulated [85].

These findings mentioned above are consistent with free radical theory of aging that free radicals regulate the aging process.

Based on the above results, in 2016, a group of Key laboratory for Molecular Enzymology and Engineering, The Ministry of Education, National Engineering Laboratory for AIDS Vaccine, School of Life Sciences, Jilin University, Changchun, China examined the *in vivo* antiaging effects of L-arginine (L-Arg. **5**) by using *C. elegans*. As a result, L-arginine (L-Arg. **5**) significantly enhanced antioxidant activity and improved resistance to environment stresses in *C. elegans*. The, strong protection against stress by L-arginine (L-Arg. **5**) might be caused by scavenging reactive oxygen species (ROS) and upregulating the expression of longevity genes, such as *heat shock protein* (*hsp*)-16.2, *superoxide dismutase* (*sod*)-3, *daf*-2 (*daf*-2 encodes a receptor tyrosine kinase that is *C. elegans* insulin/insulin-like growth factor (IGF) receptor ortholog), and *daf*-16.

This study suggested that environment stresses have long been associated with population death rate.

It was found that L-arginine (L-Arg. **5**) extends the lifespan of *C. elegans* under both oxidative and heat stress. L-Arginine (L-Arg. **5**) not only has free radical scavenging ability but also regulates the insulin/insulin-like growth factor (IGF) signaling (IlS) pathway and may be co-administered for improved stress-resistance in nematodes. L-Arginine (L-Arg. **5**) is contained in seafood, squid, shrimp, beans, eggs, peanut, wheat, garlic and others. The above findings can add to one of evidences that show the significance of the insulin/IGF signaling pathway as an ageing mechanism in *C. elegans* and potentially in humans [86].

2.5. Mitochondria and Aging

For the first time, Dr. Harman was one of the first to propose that mitochondria play a central role in ageing [87, 88].

Most of these proteins, including structural genes and assembly factors for mitochondrial proteins are encoded by nuclear DNA (nDNA). Therefore, after these proteins are synthesized by cytoplasmic ribosomes, the biosynthetic proteins must be imported into mitochondria.

Mitochondrial DNA (mtDNA) encodes only 13 subunits of oxidative phosphorylation (OXPHOS) enzyme complex (CI, III, IV and V), two ribosomal RNAs (rRNAs) and 22 transfer RNAs (tRNAs).

Expression of mitochondrial DNA (mtDNA) encoding protein and RNA species is governed by mitochondrial transcription and mitochondrial translation machinery. Protein factors (transcription factors and translation factors) are a group of proteins that specifically bind to DNA and are encoded by nuclear DNA (nDNA) [89, 90].

Mitochondria are derived from DNA double-helix of both nuclear DNA (nDNA) and mitochondrial DNA (mtDNA). Therefore, their biosynthesis in living organisms should be regulated by two DNAs of nuclear DNA (nDNA) and mitochondrial DNA (mtDNA). Mammalian mitochondria alone, including humans, are estimated to biosynthesize approximately 1500 proteins [89, 90].

2.5.1. Mitochondria and PGC-1α

The review discusses how mitochondrial dysfunction is associated with age-related diseases and what impact PGC-1α and its targets have in these diseases and their prevention.

Peroxisome proliferator-activated receptor gamma coactivator 1-alpha (PGC-1α) is a protein identified as a transcriptional coactivator that binds to the transcription factor peroxisome proliferator-activated receptor gamma (PPARγ or PPARG□, which is a nuclear receptor that is involved in insulin sensitivity and acts as a point of action for diabetes drugs. PGC-1α controls many gene expression related to energy production and heat consumption. For example, when PGC-1α is introduced into white adipocytes (having role to store fat), brown adipocyte (having role to burn fat to produce heat)-like changes such as enhanced mitochondrial biogenesis and increased expression of uncoupling protein-1 (UCP1. mitochondrial uncoupling protein. UCP 1 exists only in brown adipocytes) existing only in brown adipocytes is seen.

PGC-1α activates the transcription factor nuclear respiratory factor (NRF) 1/NRF2. NRF promotes the transcription of mitochondrial transactivation factor A (TFAM) and activates mitochondrial biogenesis.

In addition to activating mitochondrial biogenesis also in skeletal muscle, PGC-1α also induces late-phase traits such as increased fatty acid oxidation and increased type I myosin heavy chain (MHC), PGC-1α is thought to have an important function role also in transformation of skeletal muscle.

PGC-1α has multiple PGC-1α isoforms (proteins that differ in structure but have the same function) whose transcription is initiated from a new exon existing upstream of the known first exon which is structural sequence of DNA encoding nucleotide sequence of mRNA. Expression of PGC-1α isoforms increases with exercise in skeletal muscle. However, the increased expression of new PGC-1α isoforms by acute exercise depends on the new PGC-1α isoforms transcribed from these novel exons. It is thought that this increased expression of new PGC-1α isoforms controls the metabolic adaptation and the increase in heat production by exercise.

On the other hand, increased expression of PGC-1α isoforms is hardly detected by acute exercise in known PGC-1α isoforms, but it is enhanced by chronic exercise. These facts suggest that the known PGC-1 isoforms play an important functional role in the transformation of skeletal muscle by training.

Furthermore, PGC-1α expression is known to decrease in skeletal muscle of type 2 diabetic patients and obese people. Therefore, it is attracting attention that reduction of expression and dysfunction of PGC-1α may be involved in insulin resistance and obesity pathology [91].

2.5.2. Relationship between Mitochondria and PGC-1α, Aging and Life-Style Related Diseases

Mitochondrial dysfunction has been thought as one of human pathogenesis [87, 91a, 91b].

The mitochondrial dysfunction is involved in the onset and progression of life-style related diseases such as neurodegenerative disease [92, 93, 94, 95], cardiovascular diseases [96], metabolic disorders [95, 97, 98] and sarcopenia (age-related muscle wasting) [99, 100, 101, 102].

Maintaining normal mitochondrial function will be necessary for aging delay, daily calorie restriction and sirtuin gene (longevity gene) [103, 104].

Peroxisome proliferator-activated receptor (PPAR) γ coactivator α (PGC-1α) integrates regulation of mitochondrial function into the modulation of different, tissue-specific metabolic pathways and therefore links mitochondrial function to important cellular signaling pathways that ultimately control cell survival [90, 105, 106, 107, 108].

2.5.3. Relationship between Mitochondrial Biogenesis and Peroxisome Proliferator-Activated Receptor Gamma Coactivator 1-Alpha (PGC-1α)

All mitochondrial ribosomal proteins (MRPs) are the organellar counterparts of the cytoplasmic ribosomal proteins of the same species to their respective organelles (cellular organelles). When mitochondria are defective in biosynthesis of mitochondrial ribosomal proteins (MRPs), content of cytoplasmic DNA (extranuclear DNA) in conjunction is lost. The mitochondrial ribosomal proteins (MRPs) are thought to be involved in the maintenance of the mitochondrial DNA [109].

The protein content of mitochondrial ribosomes is higher when compared to that (protein content) of cytoplasmic ribosomes. The mitochondrial ribosomes are thought to contain at least 100 or more different proteins [110, 111].

Based on the above fact, in 1999, a group from Department of Biochemistry and Molecular Biology, College of Medicine, University of Florida, Florida, USA characterized mitochondrial ribosomal proteins (MRPs) in four different classes of mammals (human, mouse, rat) and compared them to both their bacterial counterpart and yeast mitochondrial counterparts.

The consensus complementary DNA (cDNA) was selected from among the various expressed sequence tag sequences identified so far, and assembled by using computer simulation (*in silico*). As a result, the putative mammalian protein sequences were characterized. These putative mammalian protein (MRP) sequences were compared to the mitochondrial ribosomal protein (MRP) sequences of the two of *E. coli* and yeast.

As a result, within the four different mammalian protein classes determined (mitochondrial ribosomal protein-L5 (MRP-L5), MRP-L7, MRP-L14, and MRP-L264), the three proteins showed significant sequence similarity to ribosomal proteins from selected sources.

However, sequence conservation (ortholog, orthology (species divergence homology) within the homologous protein) between mitochondrial ribosomal proteins (MRPs) of human mammalian origin and mitochondrial ribosomal proteins (MRPs) of yeast origin was much less when compared to sequence conservation with cytoplasmic ribosomal proteins of the same species.

Additionally, in particular, the differences of sequence conservation between these mitochondria and cytoplasm have not saved the mammalian counterparts of the *E. coli* EcoL2 ribosomal protein (MRP-L14), namely, a very important His^{229} residue specific and functional for *Escherichia coli* (*E. coli*) of *E. coli* EcoL2 sequence (accession no. Sw:rl2_ecoli) and the corresponding yeast mitochondrial RML2p MRP (multidrug resistance-associated protein) sequence (yeast RML2p MRP sequence (accession no. U18779) [112].

CONCLUSION

As long as a human being is an organism, it goes through the stages of birth, infancy, adolescence, adulthood, and death. Aging is considered is as metabolic injury due to aging process. Therefore it is natural for humans to want to delay this metabolic injury as minimally as possible in order to achieve a healthy and complete life. Here are some of the important requirements for healthy life to fulfill the human aspiration:

First, mother's diet is considered to be one of the most important requirements from fetus to new production, infants to adults. Epidemiological studies have shown that in *Dutch famine*, extreme malnutrition in the mother has a profound effect on the fetus and childbirth, *etc*. For example, newborns born from malnourished mothers during pregnancy had higher rates of stillbirths and were inferior in normal height or weight when compared to newborns from mothers who had normal nutrition. Postnatal infants and adults with poor fetal nutrition appear to have a higher incidence of lifestyle-related diseases and shorter lives than infants and adults with normal nutrition.

Normal diets are functional ingredients such as vitamins, proteins, minerals and antioxidants, as well as three major nutrients. These vitamins and proteins are one of the very important factors in judging the general physical condition of infants at birth. In fact, from epidemiological surveys, proteins of prenatal diets are involved in cross over from height of the baby at birth and birth weight to general physical health condition of neonatal at birth.

The semisessential amino acid L-arginine (L-Arg. **5**) has been considered to be a source of reactive nitric oxide (NO). However, L-arginine (L-Arg. **5**) plays an important functional role on the body's toning function in living beings and various diseases. Nonetheless, L-arginine (L-Arg. **5**) has been found to play an important role in lifestyle diseases like hypertension, diabetes, Alzheimer's disease and cancer.

Aging is a negative factor for peroxisome proliferator-activated receptor gamma coactivator 1 alpha (PGC-1α) gene expression. PGC-1α plays an important role in the control of many genes that affect a wide range of physiological functions, due to its interaction with other signal transduction pathways that control mitochondrial homeostasis and protein balance. Thus, increasing stimulation of this pathway through age-related diseases can maintain and enhance PGC-1α signaling activity and then improve other vital functions at the site of aging.

Epidemiological studies strongly suggest that a mother should have a well-balanced diet before mother conception and during pregnancy to maintain the health of mothers, fetuses and adults.

References

[1] Oparin AI. *Proiskhozhdenie zhizni* [*Origin of life*]. Izd. Moskovskii Rabochii, Moscow, Russia, 1924.

[2] (*Abiogenesis*)<https://en.wikipedia.org/wiki/Abiogenesis>.

[3] (*Abiogenesis*)<https://wired.jp/2017/05/09/how-life-began/>.

[4] (*oxygen crisis*)< https://simple.wikipedia.org/wiki/Origin_of_life>.

[5] Zimmerman L (19 October 2010). "*Must all organisms age and die?*" Massachusetts Institute of Technology School of Engineering. Archived from the original on 1 November 2010. Retrieved 5 February 2012. = <https://web.archive.org/web/20101101081710/

http:// engineering.mit.edu/ live/ news/ 1223-must-all-organisms-age-and-die>.

[6] Timothy JC, Janet BC, Yong L, Hua L, Paul IE, Wayne HG. Vital signs: racial disparities in age-specific mortality among blacks or African Americans - United States, 1999 2015. *Morbidity and Mortality Weekly Report (MMWR)* 66(17), 444-456, 2017. = <https://www.cdc.gov/mmwr/volumes/66/wr/mm6617e1.htm#contribAff>.

[7] Goldsmith TC. *An introduction to biological aging theory*. 2014. Azinet Press, Annapolis Maryland, USA.

[8] Jiaquan X, Sherry LM, Kenneth DK, Brigham B, Elizabeth A. Deaths: final data for 2016. *National Vital Statistics Reports (NVSR)* 67(5), 1-76, 2018.

[9] Comfort A. *The Biology of Senescence*, 3rd ed. 1978, Elsevier Science Ltd, Amsterdam. Holland.

[10] Comfort A. *The Biology of Senescence*, 2010, CreateSpace Independent Publishing Platform, Scotts Valley, California, USA.

[11] <https:// www.tyojyu.or.jp/ net/ kenkou-tyoju/ kenkou-undou/ shintaiteki-tokucho.html>.

[12] Michael RR, Thomas F, Joseph LG, Lee FG, Daniel EM, Margarida M, Laurence DM, Robert JSR, Parvin S. What is aging? *Front Genet* 3, Article 134, 2012. Published online 2012 Jul 20.

[13] López-Otín C, Blasco MA, Partridge L, Serrano M, Kroemer G. The hallmarks of aging. *Cell* 53(6), 1194-1217, 2013.

[14] Marsman D, Belsky DW, Gregori D, Johnson MA, Low Dog T, Meydani S, Pigat S, Sadana R, Shao A, Griffiths JC. Healthy ageing: the natural consequences of good nutrition-a conference report. *Eur J Nutr* 57(Suppl 2), 15-34, 2018.

[15] Ebbs JH, Tisdall FF, Scott WA. The influence of prenatal diet on the mother and child. *The Milbank Memorial Fund Quarterly* 20(1), 35-46, 1942.

[16] National Academies of Sciences, Engineering, and Medicine. 2017. *Nutrition across the Lifespan for Healthy Aging: Proceedings of a*

Workshop. Washington, DC, USA, The National Academies Press. doi: https://doi. org/10.17226/24735.

[17] Burke BS, Harding VV, Stuart HC. Nutrition studies during pregnancy. IV. Relation of protein content of mother's diet during pregnancy to birth length, birth weight and condition of infant at birth. *J Pediatr* 23(5), 506-515, 1943.

[18] Macy IG. Complete bibliography of publications on metabolism of women during the reproductive cycle. In: Macy IG (ed.) *Nutrition and Chemical Growth in Childhood*. Vol. 1, 402, 1942. Charles C. Thomas, Springfield, Illinois, USA.

[19] Coons CM, B1unt K. The retention of nitrogen, calcium, phosphorus, and magnesium by pregnant women. *J Biol Chem* 86, 1-16, 1930.

[20] Macy IG, Hunscher HA. Evaluation of maternal nitrogen and mineral needs during embryonic and infant development. *Am J Obstet Gynecol* 27(6), 878-888, 1934.

[21] Burke BS, Beal VA, Kirkwood SB, Stuart HC. Nutrition studies during pregnancy. *Am J Obstet Gynecol* 46(1), 38-52, 1943.

[22] Cameron CS, Graham S. Antenatal diet and its influence on still-births and prematurity. *Glasgow Med J* 142(1), 1-7, 1944.

[23] Susser M, Stein Z. Timing in prenatal nutrition: a reprise of the Dutch Famine Study. *Nutr Rev* 52(3), 84-94, 1994.

[24] Reed D (ed.). *The Epidemiology of Prematurity*, 5-15, 1977. Urban & Schwarzenberg Publisher, Vienna, Austria.

[25] Antonov AN. Children born during the siege of Leningrad in 1942. *J Pediatr* 30(3), 250-259, 1947.

[26] Sindram IS. De invloed van ondervoeding op de groei van de vrucht (The influence of famine on intrauterine growth). *Ned Tijdschr Verlosk* 45, 30-48, 1945. In Dutch.

[27] Smith CA. The effect of wartime starvation in Holland upon pregnancy and its product. *Am J Obstet Gynecol* 53(4), 599-608, 1947.

[28] McCance RA, Widdowson EM, Dean RFA, Thrussell LA. Studies on undernutrition, Wuppertal 1946-9. *Medical Research Council*

Special Report Series No. 275, London, His Majesty's Stationery Office, 1951.

[29] Tompkins WT, Mitchell R McN, Wiehl DG. Maternal and newborn nutrition studies at Philadelphia lyingin- hospital. *Maternal studies II. Prematurity and maternal nutrition. The promotion of maternal and newborn health*. New York: Milbank Memorial Fund, 1955.

[30] Darby WJ, Densen PM, Cannon RO, Bridgfort E, Martin MP, Kaser MM, Peterson C, Christie A, Frye WW, Justus K, Mclellan GS, Williams C, Ogle PJ, Hahn PF, Sheppard CW, Carothers EL, Newbill JA. The Vanderbilt cooperative study of maternal and infant nutrition. I Background. ll. Methods. Ill. Description of the sample and data. *J Nutr* 51(4), 539-563, 1953.

[31] McGanity WJ, Cannon RO, Bridgforth EB, Martin MP, Densen PM, Newbill JA, McClellian GS, Chrisite A, Peterson JC, Darby WJ. The Vanderbilt cooperative study of maternal and infant nutrition. V. Description and outcome of obstetrics sample. *Am J Obstet Gynecol* 67(3), 491-500, 1954.

[32] Thmson AM. Diet in pregnancy. 1. Dietary survey technique and nutritive value of diets taken by primigravidae. *Bri J Nutr* 12(4), 446-461, 1958.

[33] Thmson AM. Diet in pregnancy. 3. Diet in relation to the course and outcome of pregnancy. *Bri J Nutr* 13(4), 509-525, 1959.

[34] Stockard CR. Developmental rate and structural expression: An experimental study of twins, 'double monsters' and single deformities, and the interaction among embryonic organs during their origin and development. *Am J Anat* 28(2), 115-277, 1921.

[35] Buklijas T. Food, growth and time: Elsie Widdowson's and Robert McCance's research into prenatal and early postnatal growth. *Stud Hist Philos Biol Biomed Sci* 47(Pt B), 267-277, 2014.

[36] McCance RA. Food, growth, and time. *Lancet* 2(7258), 671-676, 1962.

[37] McCance RA, Widdowson EM. The determinants of growth and form. *Proc R Soc Lond B Biol Sci* 185(1078), 1-17, 1974.

[38] Dobbing J. The influence of early nutrition on the development and myelination of the brain. *Proc R Soc Lond B Biol Sci* 159, 503-509, 1964.

[39] Winick M, Noble A. Cellular response in rats during malnutrition at various ages. *J Nutr* 89(3), 300-306, 1966.

[40] Brizzee KR, Vogt J, Kharetehko X. Postnatal changes in glia neuron index with a comparison of methods of cell enumeration in the white rat. *Prog Brain Res* 4, 136-149, 1964.

[41] Zamenhof S, Van Marthens E, Margolis FL. DNA (cell number) and protein in neonatal brain: alteration by maternal dietary protein restriction. *Science* 160(3825), 322-323, 1968.

[42] Davison AN, Dobbing J. Myelination as a vulnerable period in brain development. *Br Med Bull* 22(1), 40-44, 1966.

[43] Hetzel BS, Hay ID. Thyroid function, iodine nutrition and fetal brain development. *Clin Endocrinol (Oxf)* 11(4), 445-460, 1979.

[44] Miller E, Hare JW, Cloherty JP, Dunn PJ, Gleason RE, Soeldner JS, Kitzmiller JL. Elevated maternal hemoglobin A1c in early pregnancy and major congenital anomalies in infants of diabetic mothers. *N Engl J Med* 304(22), 1331-1334, 1981.

[45] Lenke RR, Levy HL. Maternal phenylketonuria and hyperphenylalaninemia. An international survey of the outcome of untreated and treated pregnancies. *N Engl J Med* 303(21), 1202-1208, 1980.

[46] Stein ZA, Susser MW, Saenger G, Marolla FA. *Famine and human development: The Dutch hunger winter of 1944/45*. 1975, Oxford University Press, New York, USA.

[47] Stein ZA, Susser MW. Maternal starvation and birth defects. In: Hook EB (ed.), *Birth defects: Risks and Consequences*. pp. 205-220, Academic Press, New York, USA.

[48] Ravelli GP, Stein ZA, Susser MW. Obesity in young men after famine exposure *in utero* and early infancy. *N Engl J Med* 295(7), 349-353, 1976.

[49] Jones AP, Friedman MI. Obesity and adipocyte abnormalities in offspring of rats undernourished during pregnancy. *Science* 215 (4539), 1518-1519, 1982.

[50] Connolly KJ, Pharoah PO, Hetzel BS. Fetal iodine deficiency and motor performance during childhood. *Lancet* 2(8153), 1149-1151, 1979.

[51] Gruenwald P, Funakawa H, Mitani S, Nishimura T, Takeuchi S. Influence of environmental factors on foetal growth in man. *Lancet* 1(7498), 1026-1028, 1967.

[52] Winick M, Noble A. Cellular response in rats during malnutrition at various ages. *J Nutr* 89(3), 300-306, 1966.

[53] Cravioto J, DeLicardie E. Environment and nutrition deprivation in children with leaning difficulties. In: Cruickshank W, Hallahan D (eds.). *Preceptual and Learning Disabilities in Children*. vol.2. 3-102, 1975. Syracuse University Press, Syracuse, NY, USA.

[54] Stein Z, Susser M. Effects of early nutrition on neurological and mental competence in human beings. *Psychol Med* 15(4), 717-726, 1985.

[55] Ebbs JH, Tisdall FF, Scott WA. The influence of prenatal diet on the mother and child. *The Journal of Nutrition* 22(5), 515-526, 1941.

[56] Hart FB, McCollum EV, Steenbock H, Humphrey GC. *Research Bull* #17, Wisconsin Agric Exper Station, 1911.

[57] Maxwell JP, Miles LM. *Obst & Gynaec Brit Emp* 32, 433, 1925

[58] Maxwell JP, Hu CH, Turnbull HM. Foetal rickets. Part I. Clinical and pathological. *J Path* 35(3), 419-440, 1932.

[59] Tovewd G. Preventive dentistry in the preschool period and particularly during foetal life. *Dent Mag Oral Topics* 55, 299-310, 1938.

[60] Coons CM, Shiefelbusch AT, Marshall GB, Coons RR. *Oklahoma Agric & Mech College, Agric Exper Station Bull* #223, 1935.

[61] People's League of Health. Nutrition of expectant and nursing mothers: Interim Report. *Lancet* 2, 10-12, 1942.

[62] Jiangsu new medical college (ed.). *Dictionary of Chinese Traditional Medicines (Zhong Yao Da Ci Dian)*, vol.1. 190 (pp.110-

115), 2490 (pp.1227-1228), vol.2. 5099 (p.2442), Shanghai Science and Technology Publishing House, Shanghai, P.R. China, 1977. In Chinese.

[63] An JH, Vranas K, Lucke M, Inoue H, Hisamoto N, Matsumoto K, Blackwell TK. Regulation of the *Caenorhabditis elegans* oxidative stress defense protein SKN-1 by glycogen synthase kinase-3. *Proc Natl Acad Sci U S A* 102(45), 16275-16280, 2005.

[64] Wu H, Zhao Y, Guo Y, Xu L, Zhao B. Significant longevity-extending effects of a tetrapeptide from maize on *Caenorhabditis elegans* under stress. *Food Chem* 130(2), 254-260, 2012.

[65] Harman D. Aging: a theory based on free radical and radiation chemistry. *J Gerontol* 11(3), 298-300, 1956.

[66] Muller FL, Lustgarten MS, Jang Y, Richardson A, Van Remmen H. Trends in oxidative aging theories. *Free Radic Biol Med* 43(4), 477-503, 2007.

[67] Chen C, Chi YJ, Zhao MY, Lv L. Purification and identification of antioxidant peptides from egg white protein hydrolysate. *Amino Acids* 43(1), 457-466, 2012.

[68] Power O, Jakeman P, FitzGerald RJ. Antioxidative peptides: enzymatic production, *in vitro* and *in vivo* antioxidant activity and potential applications of milk-derived antioxidative peptides. *Amino Acids* 44(3), 797-820, 2013.

[69] Yu J, Hu Y, Xue M, Dun Y, Li S, Peng N, Liang Y, Zhao S. Purification and identification of antioxidant peptides from enzymatic hydrolysate of *Spirulina platensis*. *J Microbiol Biotechnol* 26(7), 1216-1223, 2016.

[70] Chaturvedi R, de Sablet T, Coburn LA, Gobert AP, Wilson KT. Arginine and polyamines in Helicobacter pylori-induced immune dysregulation and gastric carcinogenesis. *Amino Acids* 42(2-3), 627-640, 2012.

[71] Clemmensen C, Madsen AN, Smajilovic S, Holst B, Bräuner-Osborne H. L-Arginine improves multiple physiological parameters in mice exposed to diet-induced metabolic disturbances. *Amino Acids* 43(3), 1265-1275, 2012.

[72] Popolo A, Adesso S, Pinto A, Autore G, Marzocco S. L-Arginine and its metabolites in kidney and cardiovascular disease. *Amino Acids* 46(10), 2271-2286, 2014.

[73] Dioguardi FS. Clinical use of amino acids as dietary supplement: pros and cons. *J Cachexia Sarcopenia Muscle* 2(2), 75-80, 2011.

[74] Dioguardi FS. To give or not to give? Lessons from the arginine paradox. *J Nutrigenet Nutrigenomics* 4(2), 90-98, 2011.

[75] Dioguardi FS. Wasting and the substrate-to-energy controlled pathway: a role for insulin resistance and amino acids. *Am J Cardiol* 93(8A), 6A-12A, 2004.

[76] de Castro Barbosa T, Lourenço Poyares L, Fabres Machado U, Nunes MT. Chronic oral administration of arginine induces GH gene expression and insulin resistance. *Life Sci* 79(15), 1444-1449, 2006.

[77] Zhu W, Jiang W, Wu LY. Dietary L-arginine supplement alleviates hepatic heat stress and improves feed conversion ratio of Pekin ducks exposed to high environmental temperature. *J Anim Physiol Anim Nutr (Berl)* 98(6), 1124-1131, 2014.

[78] Cao W, Xiao L, Liu G, Fang T, Wu X, Jia G, Zhao H, Chen X, Wu C, Cai J, Wang J. Dietary arginine and *N*-carbamylglutamate supplementation enhances the antioxidant statuses of the liver and plasma against oxidative stress in rats. *Food Funct* 7(5), 2303-2311, 2016.

[79] Shukla J, Thakur VS, Poduval TB. Arginine: appropriate dose and delivery environment makes it an anticancer molecule. *The Open Cancer Journal* 2010, 3, 1-15, 2010.

[80] Liang H, Ren M, Habte-Tsion HM, Ge X, Xie J, Mi H, Xi, B, Miao L, Liu B, Zhou Q, Fang W. Dietary arginine affects growth performance, plasma amino acid contents and gene expressions of the TOR signaling pathway in juvenile blunt snout bream, *Megalobrama amblycephala*. *Aquaculture* 461, 1-8, 2016.

[81] Goud AP, Goud PT, Diamond MP, Abu-Soud HM. Nitric oxide delays oocyte aging. *Biochemistry* 44(34), 11361-11368, 2005.

[82] Kong X, Wang T, Li W, Tang W, Zhang D, Dong H. Exogenous nitric oxide delays salt-induced leaf senescence in cotton (*Gossypium hirsutum L.*). *Acta Physiol Plant* 38, 2016.

[83] Gusarov I, Shatalin K, Starodubtseva M, Nudler E. Endogenous nitric oxide protects bacteria against a wide spectrum of antibiotics. *Science* 325(5946), 1380-1384, 2009.

[84] Liochev SI. Free radical paradoxes. *Free Radic Biol Med* 65, 232-233, 2013.

[85] Honda Y, Honda S. The daf-2 gene network for longevity regulates oxidative stress resistance and Mn-superoxide dismutase gene expression in *Caenorhabditis elegans*. *FASEB J* 13(11), 1385-1393, 1999.

[86] Ma H, Ma Y, Zhang Z, Zhao Z, Lin R, Zhu J, Guo Y, Xu L. l-Arginine enhances resistance against oxidative stress and heat stress in *Caenorhabditis elegans*. *Int J Environ Res Public Health* 13(10), pii: E969, 2016.

[87] Harman D. The biologic clock: the mitochondria? *J Am Geriatr Soc* 20(4), 145-147, 1972.

[88] Trifunovic A. Mitochondrial DNA and ageing. *Biochim Biophys Acta* 1757(5-6), 611-617, 2006.

[89] Scarpulla RC. Transcriptional paradigms in mammalian mitochondrial biogenesis and function. *Physiol Rev* 88(2), 611-638, 2008.

[90] Wenz T. Mitochondria and PGC-1α in aging and age-associated diseases. *J Aging Res* 2011, ID 810619, 12 pages.

[91] Villena JA. New insights into PGC-1 coactivators: redefining their role in the regulation of mitochondrial function and beyond. *FEBS J* 282(4), 647-672, 2015.

[91a] Trifunovic A, Larsson NG. Mitochondrial dysfunction as a cause of ageing. *J Intern Med* 263(2), 167-178, 2008.

[91b] Lanza IR, Nair KS. Mitochondrial function as a determinant of life span. *Pflugers Arch* 459(2), 277-289, 2010.

[92] Beal MF. Mitochondria and neurodegeneration. *Novartis Found Symp* 287, 183-192; discussion 192-196, 2007.

[93] Petrozzi L, Ricci G, Giglioli NJ, Siciliano G, Mancuso M. Mitochondria and neurodegeneration. *Biosci Rep* 27(1-3), 87-104, 2007.

[94] Lezi E, Swerdlow RH. Mitochondria in neurodegeneration. *Adv Exp Med Biol* 942, 269-286, 2012.

[95] Nunnari J, Suomalainen A. Mitochondria: in sickness and in health. *Cell* 148(6), 1145-1159, 2012.

[96] Dai DF, Rabinovitch PS, Ungvari Z. Mitochondria and cardiovascular aging. *Circ Res* 110(8), 1109-1124, 2012.

[97] Sorriento D, Pascale AV, Finelli R, Carillo AL, Annunziata R, Trimarco B, Iaccarino G. Targeting mitochondria as therapeutic strategy for metabolic disorders. *Scientific World Journal* 2014 Mar 13;2014:604685. doi: 10.1155/2014/604685. eCollection 2014.

[98] Peinado JR, Diaz-Ruiz A, Frühbeck G, Malagon MM. Mitochondria in metabolic disease: getting clues from proteomic studies. *Proteomics* 14(4-5), 452-466, 2014.

[99] Picca A, Lezza AMS, Leeuwenburgh C, Pesce V, Calvani R, Bossola M, Manes-Gravina E, Landi F, Bernabei R, Marzetti E. Circulating mitochondrial DNA at the crossroads of mitochondrial dysfunction and inflammation during aging and muscle wasting disorders. *Rejuvenation Res* 21(4), 350-359, 2018.

[100] Marzetti E, Calvani R, Cesari M, Buford TW, Lorenzi M, Behnke BJ, Leeuwenburgh C. Mitochondrial dysfunction and sarcopenia of aging: from signaling pathways to clinical trials. *Int J Biochem Cell Biol* 45(10), 2288-2301, 2013.

[101] Ji LL, Kang C. Role of PGC-1α in sarcopenia: etiology and potential intervention - a mini-review. *Gerontology* 61(2), 139-148, 2015.

[102] Picca A, Calvani R, Bossola M, Allocca E, Menghi A, Pesce V, Lezza AMS, Bernabei R, Landi F, Marzetti E. Update on mitochondria and muscle aging: all wrong roads lead to sarcopenia. *Biol Chem* 399(5), 421-436, 2018.

[103] Guarente L. Sirtuins in aging and disease. *Cold Spring Harb Symp Quant Biol* 72, 483-488, 2007.

[104] Guarente L. Mitochondria--a nexus for aging, calorie restriction, and sirtuins? *Cell* 132(2), 171-176, 2008.

[105] Teyssier C, Ma H, Emter R, Kralli A, Stallcup MR. Activation of nuclear receptor coactivator PGC-1alpha by arginine methylation. *Genes Dev* 19(12), 1466-1473, 2005.

[106] Rasbach KA, Schnellmann RG. Signaling of mitochondrial biogenesis following oxidant injury. *J Biol Chem* 282(4), 2355-2362, 2007.

[107] Handschin C. The biology of PGC-1α and its therapeutic potential. *Trends Pharmacol Sci* 30(6), 322-329, 2009.

[108] Wenz T. PGC-1alpha activation as a therapeutic approach in mitochondrial disease. *IUBMB Life* 61(11), 1051-1062, 2009.

[109] Myers AM, Pape LK, Tzagoloff A. Mitochondrial protein synthesis is required for maintenance of intact mitochondrial genomes in *Saccharomyces cerevisiae*. *EMBO J* 4(8), 2087-2092, 1985.

[110] Matthews DE, Hessler RA, Denslow ND, Edwards JS, O'Brien TW. Protein composition of the bovine mitochondrial ribosome. *J Biol Chem* 257(15), 8788-8794, 1982.

[111] Graack HR, Wittmann-Liebold B. Mitochondrial ribosomal proteins (MRPs) of yeast. *Biochem J* 329 (Pt 3), 433-448, 1998.

[112] O'Brien TW, Fiesler SE, Denslow ND, Thiede B, Wittmann-Liebold B, Mougey EB, Sylvester JE, Graack HR. Mammalian mitochondrial ribosomal proteins (2). Amino acid sequencing, characterization, and identification of corresponding gene sequences. *J Biol Chem* 274(51), 36043-36051, 1999.

In: Natural Anti-Aging Plants … ISBN: 978-1-53616-282-0
Editor: Noboru Motohashi

Chapter 2

Medicinal Phytochemicals as Potent Anticancer and Antidiabetic Agents

***Roopa Naik*[1,*], *J. Seetharamappa*[1,†] *and Noboru Motohashi*[2,‡]**
[1]Department of Chemistry, Karnatak University, Dharwad, India
[2]Meiji Pharmaceutical University, Noshio Kiyose-shi, Tokyo, Japan

Abstract

Before the birth of modern medicine, ancient civilizations were using different plants to treat the common illness and a number of death causing diseases. They knew the uses of plants that were available in the nature depending on their habitat. They also knew how to use different plants strategically for the particular treatment. The World Health Organization (WHO) has stated that cancer and diabetes are the most death causing diseases in the world. According to the WHO, traditional therapy of medicine is still in practice today and about 80% of the world's population is using the plants for treating the common ailment. Diabetes is a serious chronic disorder which occurs due to increased level of sugar

* Corresponding Author's E-mail: roopanaik89@gmail.com.
† Corresponding Author's E-mail: jseetharam97@gmail.com.
‡ Corresponding Author's E-mail: noborumotohashi@jcom.home.ne.jp.

in the blood. Plant products or plants do not cause side effects to human body. Plants constitute natural materials like antioxidants, flavanoids, tannins and vitamins C and E, which are able to control the function of β-cells and help in regulating the sugar level in the blood. Herbs are able to make the human body and health stronger at very basic point. Utilization of medicinal plants for the prevention and treatment of chronic diseases is a great attempt in modern medicinal therapy. Practice of using the herbs or plant products against various physical health issues will not be trim down in the upcoming days since they are affordable as they are cheap, non-toxic, feasible and very safe to health in all aspects.

Keywords: phytochemicals, anticancer and antidiabetic agents

ABBREVIATIONS

AO/EtBr	acridine orange/ethidium bromide
DCFH-DA	2,'7'-dichlorofluorescin diacetate
DAPI	4,'6-diamino-2-phenylindoldihydrochloride
DEM	diethyl maleate
MTT	3-(4,5-dimethythiazol-2-yl)-2,5-diphenyl tetrazolium bromide
EACC	Ehrlich ascites carcinoma cell lines
FBS	fetal bovine serum
FC	Folin-Ciocalteu
GDM	gestational diabetes mellitus
GOD	glucose oxidase
IC_{50}	half maximal inhibitory concentration
HDL-C	high-density lipoprotein cholesterol
HPLC	high performance liquid chromatography
HIV	human immunodeficiency virus
IC_{50}	50% inhibitory concentration
IC_{90}	90% inhibitory concentration
LDH	lactate dehydrogenase
LC_{50}	50% lethal concentration
LC-ESI-MS/MS	liquid chromatography-ESI-mass spectrometry

LDL-C	low-density lipoprotein cholesterol
MB	methylene blue
NE mix	natural extracts mixture
ORAC	oxygen radical absorbance capacity
POD	peroxidase
PI	propidium iodide
STZ	streptozotocin
SRB assay	sulforhodamine B assay
TPC	total phenolic content
TEAC	Trolox equivalent antioxidant capacity
TBEA	trypan blue exclusion assay
VA	vinca alkaloids

1. Introduction

Plants have been an important part of our life from the beginning. From the earliest society, it is known that India is the biggest repository of herbs and medicinal plants. Plants and their products are very important to our health, growth and finally for the existence of humans. Since the origin of humans, the practice of using the plants for treating and healing some common illness has been reported. In traditional practice of medicine, a number of plants and their parts are used to treat the diseases. Increased prominence on the consumption of plants and their parts as source of medicine is mainly attributed to the increased population, insufficient supply of drugs and improved resistance power of currently available drugs against infection and so on. In modern era, scientists have faced the challenges of discovering the effective medicines for many diseases including diabetes and different types of cancer. Research work and traditional reference on different plants and their species have revealed that these have anticancer and antidiabetic activities. The scientific community has developed the new therapies and drugs against death causing diseases like cancer and diabetes using either the plants or their products. Success has been noticed in the creation of a number of staple drugs and efficient technologies for the treatment of many life threatening health problems [1].

2. Medicinal Plants

Medicinal plants are like "wealthy storage houses" of novel drugs. These drugs can be applied as main ingredients in different medicinal therapies. Chemical contents derived from the plants are natural, biodegradable or nature friendly matter and are very safe to use. These properties have drawn the attention of scientific community to explore phytochemicals and medicinal plants for the treatment of various health problems. In the field of drug discovery and design, plant products are useful due to their low toxicity, low cost, availability *etc.* International market of drugs comprises 32% of total products from plant sources with effective properties [2]. Some important uses of medicinal plants or herbs are given in Figure 1.

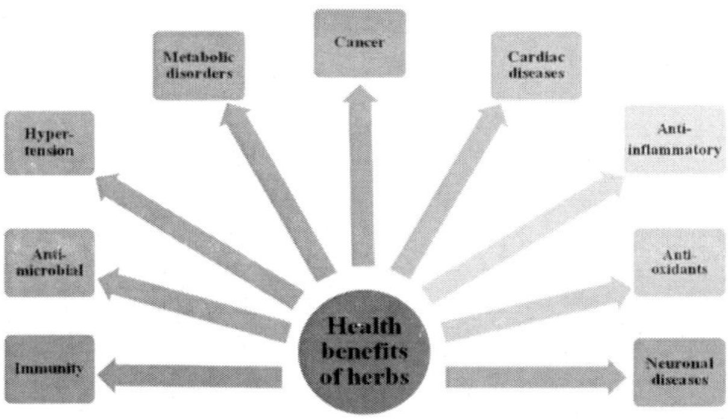

Figure 1. Important health benefits of herbs.

3. Classification of Phytochemicals of Medicinal Plants

Phytochemicals of medicinal plants can be generally divided into different classes based on the metabolites present in them. Some of the bioactive phytochemicals present in medicinal plants are tabulated in Table 2. The classification of phytochemicals is represented in Figures 2 and 3.

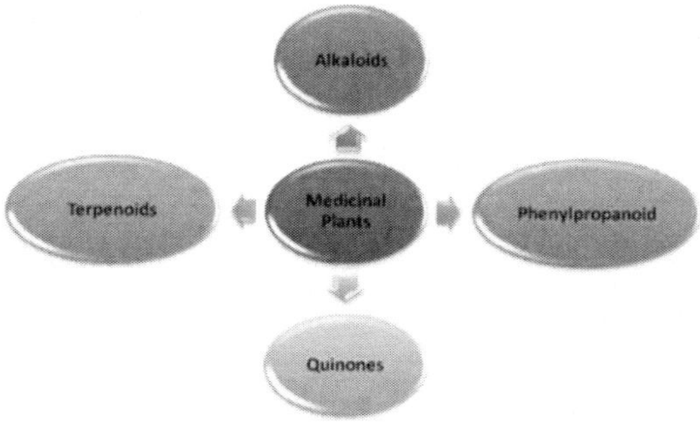

Figure 2. Classification of phytochemicals present in medicinal plants.

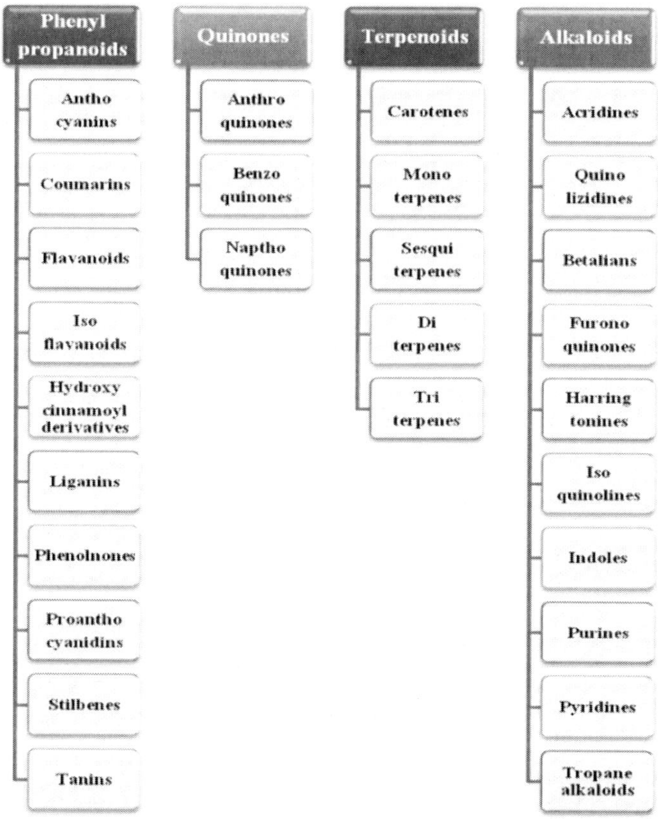

Figure 3. Subclasses of phytochemicals.

4. GENERAL PROPERTIES OF MEDICINAL PLANTS

Flow chart of isolation/extraction of phytochemicals is shown in Figure 4.

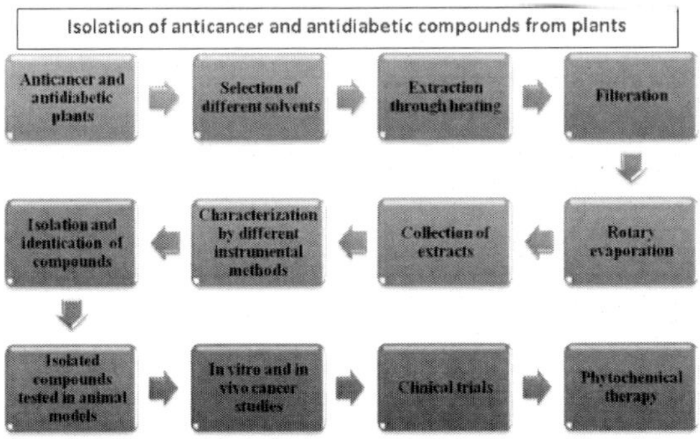

Figure 4. Flow chart showing the isolation process of anticancer/antidiabetic compounds from medicinal plants.

Let us discuss about the phytochemicals that are used in cancer phytotherapy.

5. CANCER

Cancer is a non-inherent and severe metabolic disease that occurs due to mutation of gene after birth. Cancer is the continuous and uncontrolled process of multiplication of abnormal cells in the human body. It arises due to gene mutation. Consequently, the uncontrolled condition of cell multiplication leads to tumor of malignant cells. Once the cancer cell is developed in any part of the body, it will have the ability to exterminate the normal body cells and spreads throughout the body. At present, cancer is one of the leading causes of death. The number of cancer death cases is constantly increasing around the globe. Estimated number of cases of death due to cancer by 2030 would be 21 million. It is known that over 200 different types of cancer are studied till date [3, 4]. Some types of cancer are shown in Figure 5.

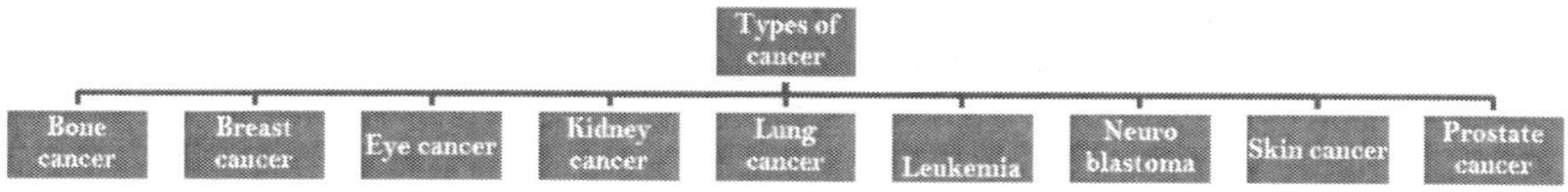

Figure 5. Various types of cancer.

Some of the cancers causing agents are listed below:

- Chemical agents or exposure to toxic compounds
- Radiation effect that causes ionization in the body
- Genetic aspects
- Some strong pathogens that result in mutation in genes [5].

A few general symptoms and signs related to the development of cancer are listed below:

- Considerable weight loss
- Fatigue
- Change in the skin color
- Pain in the body and particular part
- Change in the function of bladder
- Fever and relentless cough
- Change in the voice
- Difficulties in swallowing the food
- Continued indigestion of food
- Unusual bleeding from the excretion
- Persistent ulcers
- Changes in the size or colour of the mole on the skin
- Formation of lumps or tissue masses *etc* [6, 7].

Table 1. The list of medicinal plants with phytochemicals that fight against specific types of cancer

No.	Plant's Name	Phytochemical derived	Specific cancer type controlled
1	*Curcuma longa*	curcumin	Leukemia, glioblastoma and colon cancer, Breast, lung, colon, prostate, esophagus, liver and skin cancer
2	*Debregeasia saeneb,* *Camelia sinesis*	tannins epicatechin gallate, epicatechin, epigallocatechin	Internal tumors Lung, bladder, skin, prostate and breast cancer
3	*Peganum harmala*	harmine	Breast cancer
4	*Solanum nigrum*	solamargine, solasonine	Breast, liver, lung and skin cancer
5	*Allium wallichii*	steroids, terpenoids, flavonoids, reducing sugars and glycosides	Prostate cancer, breast cancer, cervical cancer
6	*Ginkgo biloba*	ginkgetin, ginkgolide A & B	Hepatocarcinoma, ovary, prostate, colon and liver cancer
7	*Bauhinia variegate*	kaempferol galactoside	Breast, lung and liver cancer
8	*Ziziphus spina-christi*	doxorubicin, spinanine-A, rutin, quercetin	Lung cancer and breast cancer
9	*Colchicum autumnale*	colchicin	Hodgkin's lymphoma, chronicgranulocytic leukemia
10	*Polygonum Cuspidatum*	resveratrol	Colorectal, skin and liver cancer
11	*Capsicum annuum*	luteolin	Colorectal cancer
12	*Sylibum marianum*	silibinin	Lung, liver, skin, colon andprostate cancer
13	*Vitis vinifera*	procyanidins	Human colon cancer
14	*Aloe vera*	alexin B, emodin	Leukemia, stomach cancer
15	*Annona crassiflora*	caffeic acid, sinapic acid, rutin	Glioma, renal, ovary cancer
16	*Leea indica*	gallic acid	Ehrlich ascites carcinoma
17	*Solanum lycopersicum*	lycopene	Prostate and colon cancer
18	*C. roseus*	vinblastine, vincristine	Breast, ovary, cervix, lung, rectum and testis cancer
19	*Citrus limon*	5-hydroxy-6,7,8,30,40-penta-methoxyflavone	Human colon cancer
20	*Smilax chinensis*	tannin, saponins, flavonoid	Sarcoma-180 and ascites sarcoma
21	*Pyrus malus*	quercetin, procyanidin	Colon cancer
22	*Syzygium cumini*	kaempferol-7-*O*-methylether, γ–sitosterol	Leukemia
23	*Plumbago zeylanica*	plumbagin	Blood and skin cancer

Many tests are available to screen and diagnose the cancer. Ways and protocols of treatments differ for different types of cancer and also depend on the patient's condition. But, most treatment follows the one or the other therapies in the following:

- Surgery
- Chemotherapy
- Radiation therapy

But, all these treatments have one or the other side effects including the lot of pain in surgery, bleeding, fatigue, infection *etc*. Chemotherapy may induce hair loss, vomiting, nausea, headache, muscle pain, stomach pain, sores in mouth and throat, diarrhea, constipation and blood related diseases like anemia, thrombocytopenia and leucopenia *etc*. Radiation therapy also has side effects such as sores in mouth and gum, stiffed jaw, nausea, difficulty in swallowing the food, decay of teeth, swelling in the body part called lymph edema, dryness in the mouth *etc* [8, 9, 10, 11].

Besides these, there is a need of alternative, improved and potential way of treatment and therapies for all types of cancer. In this way, the method of treatment that includes chemopreventive plant products is healthier and well suited to reduce the side effects of currently using cancer therapies. The list of phytochemicals used in the treatment of cancer is indicated in Table 1.

6. Plants for Cancer Treatment

The ongoing research around the world explores the effective therapy for the treatment of cancer. One of the best methods in practice includes the use of plants or their products to kill the cells with carcinogenic activity. Doctors and specialists prefer this type of treatment because therapies based on organics of plant may not have severe side effects as compared to that due to chemotherapy and radiation therapy.

Some plants have natural ability to suppress the spreading and risk factor of growing the different types of cancer. Around 450-470 species of plants available in nature [12] are used as remedial herbs besides using them in cancer therapy. Some examples of plants that have cancer inhibiting ability are given below:

6.1. Vinca Alkaloids

Vinca alkaloids (VAs) are isolated from periwinkle plant, *Catharanthus roseus* (*C. roseus*) that belongs to Apocynaceae family. In the scientific literature, these alkaloids are named as "monoterpenoid indole alkaloids." VAs are a resourceful phytochemicals which are used in the treatment of different types of cancer. VAs possesses cytotoxic and hypoglycemic effects. Typically, these plants can be used as medicine for diabetes, infections and high blood pressure (hypertension). In addition, these alkaloids are employed in the treatment of various cancers namely breast, liver, testicles and lung cancer. The main components of VAs in practice are vincristine, vinorelbine, vindesine and vinblastine. Recently, the derivatives of VAs (semi-synthetic products) have entered into the market. These include vinorelbine, vindesine, vinfosiltine and vinovelbine. These were tested for their anticancer activity by single administrating or in combination administration with other anticancerous agents. VAs have cytotoxic property and so, they arrest the division of cells and lead to cell death. These vincristine and vinblastine have the ability to bind to the specific site of protein called tubulin heterodimers that help in bringing the distraction among functions of microtubules or it can seize the metaphase stage of cell cycle. Microtubules play a crucial role in the division of cell; without microtubules, cell division does not occur. These VAs preoccupy the structure of functional units of tubulin and arrest the cell division [13, 14].

Vinblastine: This is a type of VAs which helps in suppressing the angiogenesis. The process through which a new blood vessel originates from the pre-existed blood vessel is called angiogenesis. This is the key step in the formation of malignant from the tumor. Hodgkin's disease (HD), non-Hodgkin's lymphoma (NHL), germ-cell tumors (GCT) and breast cancer can be treated using vinblastine [15].

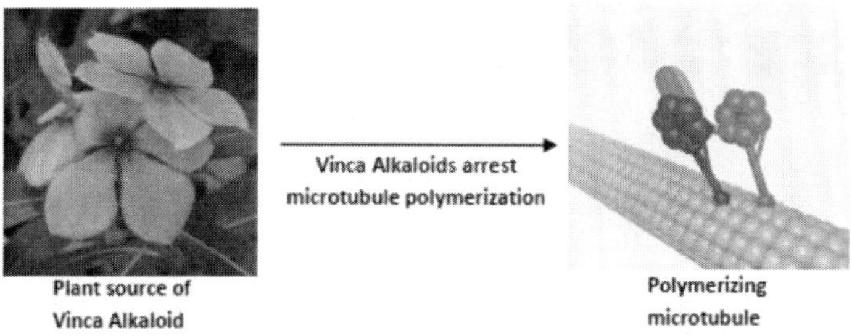

Figure 6. Illustration of the influence of vinca alkaloid on polymerization of microtubules.

Vincristine: It is used as an effective anticancer agent for several years. This has been approved as medicine to treat acute myeloid leukemia (AML), acute rhabdomyosarcoma (RMS), lymphocytic leukemia, Wilm's tumor (nephroblastoma), neuroblastoma, small cell lung cancer, Hodgkin's disease (HD) and several lymphomas. It is also named as leurocristine. Vincristine is also employed in the treatment of a number of hematologic disorders specifically non-malignant type of hematologic problems like hemolytic uremic syndrome (HUS), refractory autoimmune thrombocytopenia, and thrombotic thrombocytopenia purpura (TTP) or chronic idiopathic thrombocytopenic purpura (ITP), *etc*. The mechanism of action of vincristine is similar to that of vinblastine which binds to tubulin protein thereby arrests the separation of chromosomes at metaphase stage which leads to cell apoptosis. It also helps in suppressing the production and maturation of leukocytes.

Vinorelbine: It is used in chemotherapy. Its action is similar to that of vinblastine. This shows the signs of excellent tumor suppressing property, mainly in breast cancer, non-small cell lung cancer (NSCLC) and bone cancer patients. Besides these, it is used to reduce the lipid bilayer membranes. It is a semisynthetic derivative of VAs. This has been approved as a chemotherapeutic agent in USA for the treatment of multiple cancers.

6.2. *Tinospora cordifolia* (Wile) Miers

Tinospora cordifolia (*T. cordifolia*) is commonly called as guduchi or giloya or heartleaf moon seed plant. *T. cordifoliais* is termed as "amrita" since it has the ability to introduce liveliness, youthfulness and prolonged existence. A particular part of *T. cordifolia* is employed as a medicinal agent for general illness such as vomiting, anemia, piles, chronic fever, urinary tract infections (UTIs), weakness, fever, indigestion, jaundice and even acts as an antidote for snake bite. Its extract can be also used in the

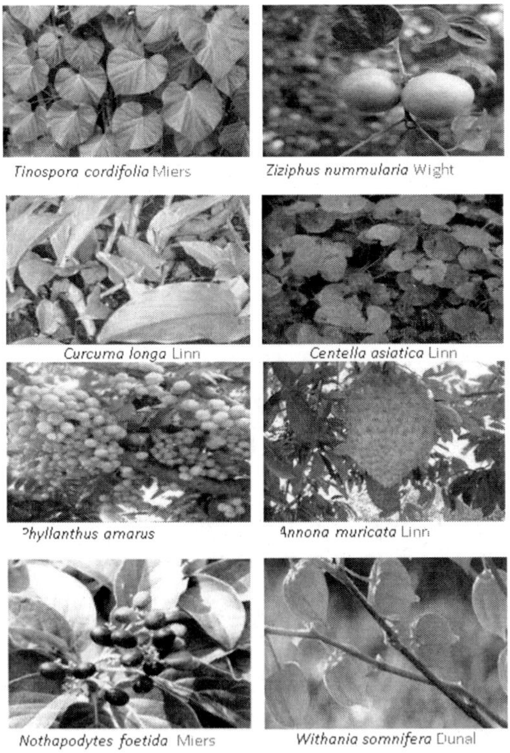

Figure 7. A few anticancer activity exhibiting plants.

treatment of skin diseases. Besides these interesting properties, *T. cordifolia* possesses immune modulatory, adaptogenic, anti-inflammatory, anti-allergic, anti-arthritic and antioxidant properties. The methanol extracts of different parts of this plant consist of phenyl propanoids, nor-diterpene furan glycosides, choline, tinosporin, columbin, isocolumbin, palmatine, tetrahydropalmatine, magnoflorine diterpene furan glycosides, phytoecdysones, *etc* [16, 17, 18]. *T. cordifolia* showed excellent anticancer activity towards HeLa cells *in vitro* thereby revealing that the extract obtained from *T. cordifolia* could be used as a potent anticancer agent. Some important plants with anticancer activity are shown in Figure 7.

7. Diabetes

Diabetes is one of the life hindering and dangerous ailment which is classified as insulin-dependent and non-insulin dependent diabetes. It is very common metabolic disorder widespread around the world. It mainly affects the fundamental biochemical pathways and biological functions in the human body. It can be found in every human age group. Imperfection in the secretion of insulin and/or action of secreted insulin in the diabetic problem leads to hyperglycemia. In conventional therapy, exogenous insulin is used to treat insulin-dependent diabetes while non-insulin dependent diabetes is cured by synthesized hyperglycemic agents. Most of the times, synthetic agents cause adverse effects on health of patients. To avoid these side effects of synthetic drugs, scientists have started to study the traditional knowledge that uses natural herbs for the treatment of many ailments. They have been historically applied in the treatment of diabetes worldwide since natural herbs do not cause any side effects. Most of the drugs available in the market are obtained from plants by direct or indirect methods. Diabetes results in various health issues that include:

- Diseases related to teeth and gum
- Loss of sight and eye problems

- Problems in foot like numbness, ulcers in/on the body and untreated wounds
- Heart disease (cardiac disease)
- Diabetic neuropathy by damaged nerves
- Stroke
- Kidney disease including retention of water in the body and failure of kidney, *etc*

General symptoms of diabetes are indicated below:

- Augmented thirsty level and urination
- Frequent hungriness
- Increased tiredness
- Blurriness in the vision
- Feel deadness or itchiness in the feet or hands
- Takes long time to heal the wounds compared to earlier times
- Inexplicable weight loss

We can observe some of the symptoms in type 1 diabetes in earlier days but for type 2 diabetes symptoms developed very slowly (it may take several years) compared to type 1 diabetes.

7.1. Types of Diabetes

There are three types of diabetes. They are type 1 diabetes, type 2 diabetes and gestational diabetes mellitus (GDM).

Type 1 diabetes: Other name of type I diabetes is juvenile diabetes which arises due to the failure of the body to produce insulin. This type of patients are insulin-dependent, hence they must take artificial insulin for the daily survival.

Type 2 diabetes: It mainly affects the pathway of utilization of insulin by the body. The body produces insulin but efficiency of cells to respond to insulin that is produced is declined compared to earlier process. Type 2 diabetes is very common worldwide and it is correlated with the obesity of the person.

Table 2. Some herbal plants having antidiabetic actions

No.	Botanical Name	Common Name	Part Used	Active Constituent
1	*Aegle marmelos*	Bael	Leaf	aegelin
2	*Allium cepa*	Onion	Bulb	quercetin
3	*Azadirachta indica*	Neem	Bark and leaf	quercetin, rutin, nimbidin
4	*Brassica juncea*	Indian mustard	Seed	isothiocyanate glycosidesingrin
5	*Cajanus cajan*	Pigeonpea	Leaves	Two globulins, cajanin and concajanin
6	*Eucalyptus globules*	Blue gum	Leaves	polyphenols, proanthocyanidins, anthocyanins
7	*Aloe vera*	Aloe	Leaves	barbaloin
8	*Catharanthus roseus*	Madagascar periwinkle	Leaves	indole alkaloid (vincristine)
9	*Cryptolepis Sanguinolenta*	Anantmul	Stem	cryptolepine
10	*Olea europia*	Olive leaf	Leaf	oleuropeoside

Gestational diabetes mellitus (GDM): It arises mainly in women all through pregnancy period. In this condition, the body becomes weak to respond to insulin. It can be found in a few women but not in all during the pregnancy period. It generally resolves after the birth of a baby.

Besides this monogenic diabetes, cystic fibrosis-related diabetes (CFRD) may be developed. It is less common type of diabetes [19, 20].

Some parts of the plants/plants used in the treatment of diabetes are *Acacia arabica*, *Achyranthes aspera*, *Acosmium panamense*, *Aegle marmelose*, *Allium sativum*, *Aloe barbadensis* Miller, *Andrographis paniculata*, *Annona squamosa*, *Argyreia nervosa*, *Artemisia herba*, *Averrhova bilimbi*, *Azadirachta indica*, *Barleria prionitis*, *Biophytum sensitivum*, *Brassica nigra*, *Bryonia alba*, *Caesalpinia bonducella*, *Cajanus cajan*, *Carum carvi*, *Casearia esculenta*, *Chamaemelum nobile*,

Table 3. Medicinal plants/parts of plants used as antidiabetic/hypoglycemic/hyperglycemic agents

No.	Plant Name	Part of the plant Used	Activity	References
1	*Alangium lamarckii*	Leaves	Antidiabetic	[23]
2	*Axonopus compressus*	Leaves	Antidiabetic	[24]
3	*Albizia odoratissima*	Barks	Antidiabetic	[25]
4	*Brassssica juncea*	Seed	Hypoglycemic	[26]
5	*Berberis vulgaris*	Root	Hypoglycemic	[27]
6	*Caesalpinia digyna*	Root	Antidiabetic	[28]
7	*Centaurium erythrea*	Leaves	Antidiabetic	[29]
8	*Chaenomeles sinensis*	Fruits	Antidiabetic	[30]
9	*Catharanthus roseus*	Leaves	Hypoglycemic	[31]
10	*Costus speciosus*	Rhizome	Antidiabetic	[32]
11	*Cyclocarya paliurus*	Bark	Hypoglycemic	[33]
12	*Cocos nucifera*	Leaves	Anti-hyperglycemic	[34]
13	*Hybanthus enneaspermus*	Whole plant	Antidiabetic	[35]
14	*Lithocarpus polystachyus*	Leaves	Hypoglycemic	[36]
15	*Marrubium vulgare*	Aerial part	Hyperglycemia	[37]
16	*Ocimum sanctum*	Aerial part	Antidiabetic	[38]
17	*Semecarpus anacardium*	Nut milk	Antidiabetic	[39]
18	*Symplocos cochinchinensis*	Leaves	Antidiabetic	[40]
19	*Zygophyllum album*	Whole plant	Antidiabetic	[41]
20	*Vaccinium arctostaphylos*	Fruits	Antidiabetic	[42]
21	*Holarrhena pubescens*	Seeds	antihyperlipidemic	[43]
22	*Eucalyptus globules*	Leaves	Antidiabetic	[44]
23	*Dioscorea oppositifolia*	Roots	Antidiabetic	[45]
24	*Boerhaavia diffusa*	Roots and leaves	Antidiabetic	[46]
25	*Bougainvillea spectabilis*	Leaves	Antidiabetic	[47]
26	*Bauhinia purpurea*	Leaves	antihyperlipidemic	[48]
27	*Alangium salvifolium*	Leaves	Antihyperlipidemic and antihyperglycemic	[49]
28	*Radix rehmanniae*	Rhizomes	Antidiabetic	[44]
29	*Pterocarpus marsupium*	Bark	Antidiabetic	[50]
30	*Mucuna pruriens*	Seed	Antidiabetic	[51]

Cichorium intybus, *Citrulus colocynthis*, *Coriandrum sativum*, *Dorema aucheri*, *Eclipta alba*, *Helicteres isora*, *Mangifera indica*, *Myrcia bella*, *Momordica charantia*, *Syzygium cumini*, *Gymnema sylvestre*, *Trigonella foenum-graecum*, *Tinospora cordifolia*, *Ocimum tenuiflorum*, *Aegle marmelos*, *Phyllanthus emblica*, *etc*. All these plants are well participated in some of the important action mechanisms like improving the secretion of insulin, reduction of glucose absorption capacity of intestine, enhancement of the glucose absorption by tissues and muscles and also inhibition of the production of glucose from liver cells [21, 22].

The structures of phytochemicals having antidiabetic activity are shown in Figure 8 below:

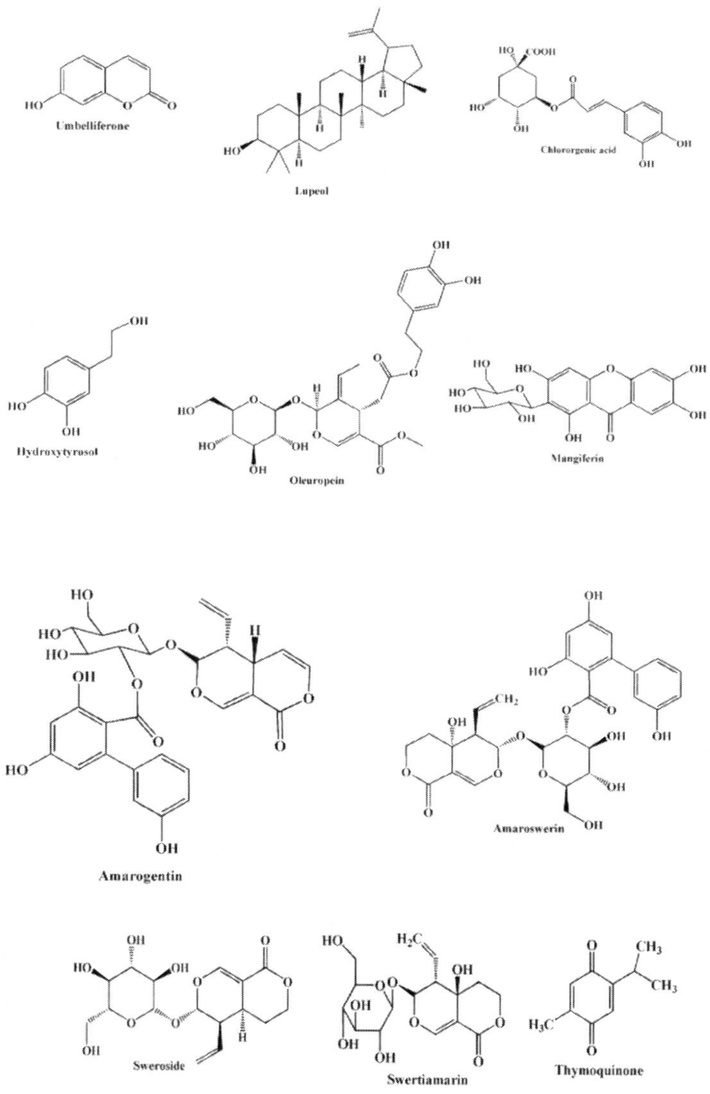

Figure 8. (Continued).

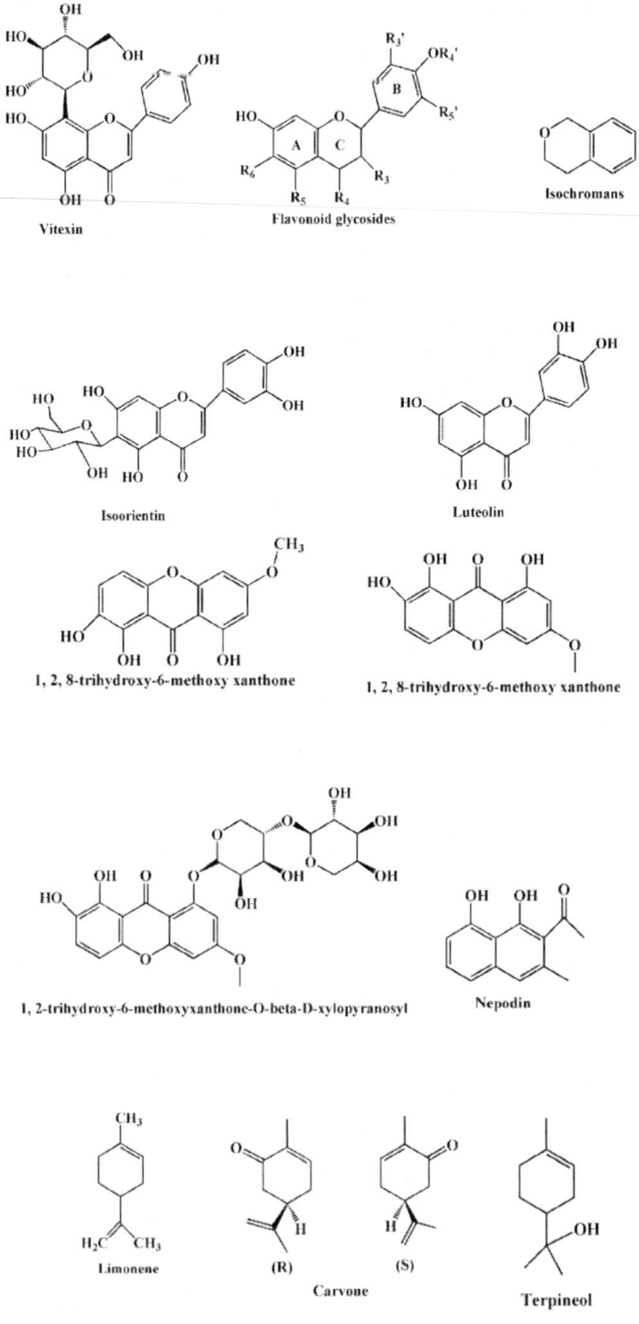

Figure 8. (Continued).

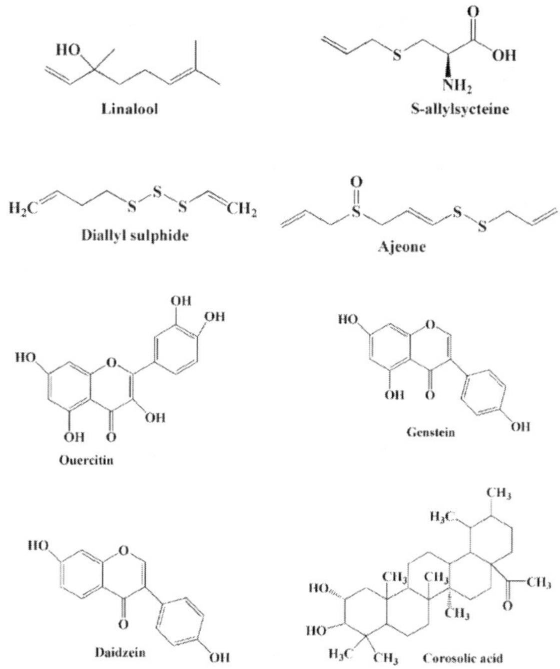

Figure 8. Some of the phytochemicals that exhibit antidiabetic activity.

8. Isolation, Characterization and Applications of Anticancer and Antidiabetic Plants

8.1. Anticancer Properties

Peperomia pellucida is a Malaysian plant commonly called as 'Ketumpangan air.' This plant is used as a multifunctional medicinal plant in different regions. Different parts of this plant and its decoction are used in the treatment of bone aches and pains, headache, eczema, abdominal pains, mental disorder and fever, against hemorrhage, as cholesterol and uric acid reducing agent and also for renal problem. Leaf extract of *Peperomia pellucida* was used by Wei and coworkers to analyze the composition of chemical content and anticancer activity [52]. They have isolated the leaf extract using 70% methanol with a concentration limit of 1 mg/mL. In order to determine the chemical composition of leaf extract, the investigators have employed gas chromatograph-mass spectrometer (GC-MS). The contents of test solution were spotted out by their spectra. The findings of this study confirmed that the phytol was the major diterpene compound which contributed towards anticancer property of leaf extract. Besides this, (9Z,12Z)-9,12-octadecadienoic acid and methyl ester were present in the extract. They also exhibited the anticancer activity. In order to determine the anticancer property, the investigator has used colorimetric MTT (3-(4,5-dimethythiazol-2-yl)-2,5-diphenyl tetrazolium bromide) assay and tested for 48 hr proliferation towards cell lines of human breast adenocarcinoma (MCF-7). Cancer cells grown in 5% CO_2 atmosphere with standard cell medium of RPMI 1640 that was supplemented with 5% fetal bovine serum (FBS) were taken to confirm the anticancer activity. Very sharp decrease in the viability of cancer cells (up to 54%) was noticed when the concentration of test solution was 30 μg/mL. Half maximal inhibitory concentration (IC_{50}) was observed to be 10.4 ± 0.06 μg/mL. The phytochemical contents of methanol extract of the leaf used in the present study showed good anticancer activity. Results of the present study suggested that methanol extract of *Peperomia pellucida* leaf was a potential medicinal drug for the treatment of breast cancer.

People use *Saururus chinensis* plant extract and its parts as diuretic and as a detoxifying agent for the treatment of diseases like edema, jaundice, gonorrhoea and several other inflammatory conditions, especially in India and China. The interesting point about this plant is that it possess multifunctional activities such as anti-inflammatory, antidiabetic, antioxidant, anticarcinogenic, hepato-protective, nephro-toxic, neuroprotective activity, carcinogenic and mutagenic properties. Alaklabi and coworkers [53] have evaluated the anticancer activity in *Saururus chinensis* (*S. chinensis)* root extracts. In order to determine the chemical contents of the root extract of *S. chinensis*, they have used ethyl acetate, methanol, ethanol and water extracts. The investigators have determined the total phenolic and flavonoid content present in the samples of dried root using the assay methods like Folin-Ciocalteu reagent (FC reagent) and aluminium chloride by colorimetry. Cancer cell viability test was performed using MCF-7 cell lines by MTT assay method by following the US National Cancer Institute (NCI) protocol to confirm the anticancer activity. The compounds of root extract were analyzed for primary anticancer assay that is mainly towards human breast cancer by performing MTT assay. Extracts of compounds from water, ethyl acetate, methanol and ethanol were tested. Results of *in vitro* screening unravel that the compounds extracted in water possessed excellent anticancer activity in comparison with MCF-7 cell lines. These results showed that 54.2% inhibition was observed at a test sample concentration of 100 μg/mL. Finally, the compound extracted from the root of *S. chinensis* in water medium exhibited greater anticancer activity. Further, it showed stronger fatal effect on human breast cancer cells such as MCF-7 cell lines. Other compounds extracted in ethyl acetate, methanol and ethanol showed lower anticancer potency towards MCF-7 cell lines.

Mishra and coworkers have isolated the *Betula utilis (B. utilis)* bark, characterized and screened it for anticancer activity [54]. *B. utilis*is also known as Himalayan silver birch and Bhojpatra. It is employed as a traditional medicine for human immunodeficiency virus (HIV), renal, inflammation and bladders and also for the treatment of cancer. The plant bark is employed in the Ayurvedic medicine for the treatment of a number of diseases, since it possess activities like carminative, antiseptic, contraceptive, *etc.* According to literature, the bark contains acetyl oleanolic acid, lupeol, betulinic acid, betulin, oleanolic acid, lupenone, sitosterol, methyl betulate and karachic acid. In this study, the investigators have used methanol to extract the phytochemicals present in the bark of *B. utilis* and then fractionated using different solvents (*n*-hexane, chloroform, ethyl acetate and *n*-butanol and water). The samples obtained by different extractions were primarily screened for cytotoxic activity using different types of cell lines that exhibited cancer property by sulforhodamine B assay (SRB assay). The human cancer cell lines employed in this investigation for *in vitro* anticancer activities are A172-glioblastoma, MCF-7-Breast adenocarcinoma, BxPC-3-Pancreatic adenocarcinoma, DLD-1 colorectal adenocarcinoma, PLC/PRF/5 human hepatoma cell line, SK-OV-3 human ovarian carcinoma, A549 lung carcinoma, DU-145 prostate carcinoma and Caki-1 renal cell carcinoma. The results of anticancer activity screening of samples of bark extract showed that the extracts of methanol, ethyl acetate and chloroform have excellent potency against cancer cell lines.

Vemuri *et al.* [55] have studied the ability of aqueous natural extracts mixture (NE mix) of common spices like turmeric, ginger and garlic. These common spices are mainly used for cooking in India which contain bioactive compounds like curcumin (*Curcuma longa* L., commonly called as turmeric), allicin (*Allium sativum* L. common name garlic), 6-gingerol and oleoresin (*Zingiber officinale R.* commonly named ginger). This study investigated the free radical scavenging and anti-cancer property of common species towards human breast cancer cell lines (examples - MCF-7, ZR-75-1 cells and MDA-MB-231 cells). The investigators have used the compound obtained from plants to overcome the side effects of synthetic anticancer drugs. They have tried the combinational therapeutic methods to treat different types of cancer. Tamoxifen drug is used along with natural extract mixture obtained from turmeric, ginger and garlic. Qualitative analysis of turmeric, ginger and garlic was carried out to determine the bioactive constituents. Liquid chromatography-ESI-mass spectrometry (LC-ESI-MS/MS) was employed to analyze the biologically active components of the sample. Culture of human breast adenocarcinoma MCF-7 cells and MDA-MB-231 melanoma cells was done in T-25 cell culture flask. A few different breast cancer cell lines such as MCF-7, ZR-75 and MDA-MB-231 were employed to evaluate the proliferative ability of aqueous NE mix. It was observed that the NE mix persuaded apoptosis of cancer cells. Detachments of cells were noticed in the underlying layer after 42 hr indicating the death of cancer cells. Anticancer activity was quite significant against MCF-7 and ZR-75 compared to that against MDA-MB-231. Effect of apoptosis was more pronounced for the sample that contained NE mix and tamoxifen when compared to that contained either NE mix or tamoxifen alone. This investigation revealed that aqueous natural extracts of common spices used in cooking stimulated the death of cancer cells and reduced the division of cells. In addition, the data obtained by this research indicated the possible sensitization of cancer cells by natural extract when compared to that of tamoxifen. Further study helped in developing a good anticancer agent to treat the breast cancer.

Yen and coworkers have focused on the properties of roots of *Ficus beecheyana (F. beecheyana)* (FB). They have examined the anticancer and antioxidant properties of the ethanolic and aqueous extracts of roots of *F. beecheyana* (EERFB and AERFB) [56]. The rhizomes are used as traditional medicine for diabetes and rheumatism. The present investigation utilized four different human cancer cell lines such as AGS human gastric adenocarcinoma cells, SW 872 human liposarcoma cells, HL-60 human leukemia cells, and HepG2 human hepatoma cells. In addition to the anticancer properties of root extract of FB, the investigators have also evaluated and found out the antioxidant activity of EERFB and AERFB mainly based on the oxygen radical absorbance capacity (ORAC), total phenolic content (TPC) and Trolox equivalent antioxidant capacity (TEAC). High performance liquid chromatographic (HPLC) method was employed to determine the key antioxidant contents of both ethanolic and aqueous extracts of the sample. Gallic acid, *p*-hydroxybenzoic acid, caffeic acid, chlorogenic acid, *p*-coumaric acid, and rutin were found in the extracts of root of *F. beecheyana*. All these phenolic compounds present in the sample of plant root possessed the antioxidant, antithrombosis, antiinflammatory, anti-HIV-1, and anticancer activities. Antiproliferative study of EERFB and AERFB was investigated in different human cancer cell lines both *via* intrinsic and extrinsic trails. Influence of EERFB and AERFB was tested on the cell viability of cancer cell lines. The results suggested that EERFB exhibited a stronger inhibitory effect on the development of cancer cell compared to that of AERFB. Growth of cancer cells was suppressed due to the arrest of cell cycle. Thus, EERFB was taken for further examination. The mode of apoptosis was determined. For this, EERFB treated with HL-60 cells was analyzed by flow cytometry. Current study revealed that the EERFB invaded the arrest of cell cycle of HL-60 human cancer cells through mitochondria-dependent path when compared to AERFB.

Morus nigra L. (*M. nigra*) plant was examined for antiproliferative and apoptotic effect against prostate cancer cells by Turan *et al.* [57]. This is employed in the treatment of urinary incontinence, depression, fever, dizziness, sore throat and cancer in traditional therapy. Fruits of *M. nigra* plant are rich in phenolic compounds like flavonoids, anthocyanins and carotenoids. We found from the several reports that these phenolic compounds of *M. nigra* also exhibited good antioxidant and anticancer characteristics. A number of studies on *M. nigra* have demonstrated the anticancer activity through apoptosis on human colorectal carcinoma cell line (SW480), human cervical cancer (HeLa) cell line and other types of carcinoma. The investigators have studied *in vitro* cytotoxic effects of *M. nigra* extract on prostate cancer cells. Maceration method was used for the extraction of active constituents from *M. nigra* plant materials. This study also evaluated the composition of phenolic compounds, antioxidant and antiproliferative properties. Reference anticancer agent used for testing the cytotoxic effect on prostate cancer cell lines was cisplatin. Human prostate adenocarcinoma of type PC-3, ATCC-CRL-1435 cancer cells and human normal foreskin fibroblast cells, ATCCCRL-2522 were used in the antiproliferative experiments. From the results of antiproliferative tests, it was clear that the cell cycle of PC-3 cancer cells was obstructed when a 90% inhibitory concentration (IC_{90}) concentration of diethyl maleate (DEM) was added. Both G_0 and G_1 phases of cell cycle were found to be arrested and also considerably reduced cells were noticed at the S phase. Thus, present findings are fundamental in developing an efficient anticancer agent. Active components of extract of *M. nigra* such as ascorbic acid, lectin, gallic acid and chlorogenic acid were able to snatch cell cycle at any stage which was mainly reliant on the nature of cancer cells.

Annona muricata (*A. muricata*) is used as a source plant and its components are tested for *in vitro* anticancer ability [58]. *A. muricata* is extensively used in many countries for the conventional treatment of cancer. It is also commonly named as Graviola or sour sop, which comes under the family, *Annonaceae*. Some previous research articles have revealed the anti-hyperlipidemic, anti-hyperglycemic, antimalarial, insecticidal, anti-parasitic, antibacterial, molluscicidal, antiviral and anticancer activities. Two different solvents (water and ethanol) were used to extract the phytochemicals from the leaves of *A. muricata.* The samples were screened by standard qualitative methods and the results indicated the presence of phytochemicals like terpenoids, flavanoids, saponins, coumarins and lactones, tannins, cardiac glycosides, phytosterols, anthraquinones and phenols. In the present study, the extracts of *A. muricata* leaves were screened for *in vitro* anticancer activity against tumor cell lines, namely Ehrlich ascites carcinoma cell lines (EACC). Trypan blue exclusion assay (TBEA) method was used to explore the anticancer property against EACC. The investigators have detected minimal anticancer ability with 32.9% cell death at the ethanolic extract concentration of 250 μg/mL. Besides this, at 750 μg/mL concentration 100% cell arrest was noticed, but no consequences about cell death were noticed with water extract. For ethanolic extract, 50% inhibitory concentration (IC_{50}) of 335.85 μg/mL was noticed. These findings revealed that no harmful (cytotoxic) effect was noticed on normal cells. To analyze the anticancer ability of the extract against breast cancer cell line like MDA-MB-231 (human breast adenocarcinoma cell line) and *SK-BR-3* human breast cancer cell line, MTT testing method was performed. The results of anticancer activity suggested maximum anticancer activity for ethanolic extracts against all three cell lines (EACC, MDA, and SKBR3). In order to confirm the cytotoxicity of ethanolic extract, spleen cells were taken and tests were conducted by trypan blue exclusion assay (TBEA). The results suggested the effective anticancer activity of ethanolic extract *A. muricata.* Leaves of *Zea mays* were utilized as key source for the study of an anticancer activity against Hep2 cells and were investigated by Balasubramanian and Padma [59]. Evaluation of different extracts of *Z. mays* leaves *viz.* methanol, chloroform and aqueous extract is discussed. Common name of *Z. mays* is makkacholam or maize which belongs to Gramineae family. Results of preliminary studies on aqueous, chloroform and methanol extracts of leaves disclosed strong antioxidant properties of *Z. mays.* Different tests such as viability assays (MTT assay), and Giemsa staining, propidium iodide (PI), 4,'6-diamino-2'-phenylindole dihydrochloride (DAPI), acridine orange/ethidium bromide (AO/EtBr) and EtBr staining methods were employed to study the apoptotic results upon oxidant treatment. Analysis of phytochemical disclosed that leaves of *Z. mays* consisted of phenolics and flavanoids as main components. Degree of cell demise was quantified by sulforhodamine B (SRB) and MTT assay and was performed in cells of group treated with bare H_2O_2, bare plant extract and also to combination of both H_2O_2 and plant extract. Nuclear fragmentation and anticancer ability of extracts were also investigated. From these studies, it was confirmed that extracts of leaf itself acted as apoptosis inducer in Hep2 cells. The investigators have observed better apoptotic effects mainly in aqueous and chloroform extracts. The outcome of DAPI test signified that cells with nuclear changes was more upon H_2O_2 addition and showed apoptotic ratio of 0.92. Observed results suggested that the treatment of both H_2O_2 and leaf extract triggered cytotoxicity in cancer cell lines. Compared to chloroform extract, both aqueous and methanolic extracts of leafs of *Z. mays* that was treated with oxidatively stressed cancer cells, confirmed cytotoxicity in H_2O_2-treated groups of cells. Tests on aqueous and methanol leaf extracts signified that no characteristic changes were observed in the cytotoxic action of H_2O_2 in the cancer cells. Thus, it confirmed the potential anticancer activity of *Z. mays* leaves and so could be utilized in various apoptosis related trials. Finally, the investigators observed better anticancer activity with methanolic extract compared to that with aqueous and chloroform extracts.

In vitro anticancer activity of leaf extract of *Leea indica* (*L. indica*) was evaluated by Ghagane and coworkers [60]. In the present work, the investigators have described the analysis of phytochemical constituents, antioxidant and anticancer activities of leaf extracts of *L. indica.* Soxhlet extraction method was used to get the leaf extract and different solvents (with their increasing order of polarity) such as ethyl acetate, methanol, chloroform, ethanol and water were used to prepare extract. Qualitative tests were also performed to determine phytochemical constituents present in chloroform, ethyl acetate, methanol, ethanol, and aqueous extract. Main aim of this work was to find out the anticancer activity of leaf extract. Based on the findings of phytochemical analysis, methanol, ethanol, and aqueous extracts of leaf were subjected to *in vitro* anticancer activity. DU-145 and PC-3 human prostate cancer cell lines were utilized to evaluate antiproliferative action of the extract. For this, MTT assay was performed on all the extracts. Mitochondrial dehydrogenase induced reduction of MTT by purple formazan product. In recent research, MTT assay became an *in vitro* model system. It was performed to quantify the cytotoxic effects of different substances and also of plant extracts towards cancer cell lines. Findings of MTT assay showed that methanol and ethanol extracts of leaves of *L. indica* reduced the percent sustainability of cancer cells at different level. More cytotoxic activity was noticed for methanol and ethanol extracts against cancer cell lines DU-145 and PC-3. On the other side, cytotoxic effect was null to noncancerous normal cells of mice embryo fibroblast (MEF-L929) cell line. Paclitaxel is a standard chemotherapeutic drug, which is in practice for treating the prostate cancer. Anticancer effect of the extract of *L. indica* leaves was analogous to that of paclitaxel. All these results suggested that the extract of *L. indica* could act as an effective agent and so could be utilized in the therapy of prostate cancer.

Venugopal and Liu have investigated the importance of resveratrol and ursolic acid in diet to prevent the breast cancer [61]. Resveratrol, phytoalexin, ursolic acid, and a penta-cyclic triterpenoid have taken lead in the research of medicinal field. It is present in red wine and a number research articles have confirmed about its cardioprotective effects, anticancer, antidiabetic, antiaging and antiinflammatory, neuroprotective actions. Ursolic acid found in cranberries, apples and other fruits also exhibits good anticancer property, reduces obesity along with burning of calories. Anticancer actions of both resveratrol and ursolic acid were studied by animal model, epidemiological and clinical trials. Resveratrol showed antiproliferative properties towards MCF-7 breast cancer cells, in which dose-dependent suppression of cell growth was observed. Arrest of cell cycle at S phase resulted lower concentration of resveratrol. Attendance of condensed chromatin and sub-G1 fractions were confirmed by the apoptosis induced by resveratrol and thereby inhibiting the growth of cancer cells. Even synthesized resveratrol exhibited similar apoptosis and antiproliferative effect when tested against estrogen receptor (ER)-positive (ER^+) and estrogen receptor (ER)-negative (ER^-) breast cancer cell lines. Three cell lines namely KPL-1 human breast cancer cells and MCF-7 sublines were used to understand the effect on ER+ and MKL-F human breast cancer cell lines for ER−. In case of ER+ cell lines KPL-1 and MCF-7, low concentration (<4 and 22 μmol/L, respectively) of resveratrol produced antiproliferative actions but at higher concentration of resveratrol (<44 μmol/L) cell growth of all three cell lines was suppressed. Proliferation of ER negative breast cancer cell line, MDA-MB-468 was also suppressed by resveratrol. Estrogen receptor antagonist action of resveratrol was noticed which highlighted the mechanism of cell production inhibition.

Leaves and roots of *Pandanus Odoratissimus* f. ferreus (*P. ferreus*) were examined for the dose-dependent *in vitro* anticancer property [62]. Methanol (MEPO) and water (AEPO) were used as solvents to prepare the extract of dried parts of roots and leaves. *Pandanus odoratissimus* f. ferreus belongs to the family of *Pandanaceae* copiously distributed in India. Leaves of this plant are used in Ayurveda, Unani and Siddha methods of medicine. They are used in the treatment of epilepsy, wound healing, indigestion, backache, loss of appetite, constipation, rheumatic diseases (RA), nervous system disorders, skin diseases, diabetes, infertility, urinary disorders, fever, *etc*. Steroids, glycosides, tannins and flavonoids, saponins and terpenoids are found in the methanolic extract of *P. odoratissimus.* The paste prepared using sugar and *P. odoratissimus* was used for cancer therapy in Ayurveda. *In vitro* cytotoxic and antimitotic screening assay (brine shrimps were used) and onion root tip methods were carried out on prepared extracts. Calu-6 (non-small cell lung cancer cell lines), WI (lung fibroblast cell lines) and PBMC (peripheral blood mononuclear cells) were employed to analyze the activities of both methanol and aqueous extracts by MTT assay and flow cytometric exploration. Results of cytotoxic and antimitotic assay signified the excellent actions of AEPO. It exhibited 100% lethal effect on brine shrimps at a concentration of 80 μg/mL. When compared to lethal concentration (LC_{50}) value of synthetic standard podophyllotoxin (4.16 μg/mL), AEPO was 8-fold efficient with LC_{50} value of 33.33 μg/mL. Investigators have observed 3% mitotic index for AEPO at a concentration of 10 mg/mL while it was 4% for standard cyclophosphamide. This indicated substantial antimitotic actions of AEPO. Hence, cell proliferation of calu-6 was suppressed (56-35%) when 200 μg/mL of AEPO was added in the treatment for about 24-48 hr. No significant effect of AEPO was observed on cell lines of both PBMC and WI−38. These findings clearly suggested that AEPO exhibited excellent antiproliferative actions and hence it could be used as an anticancer agent.

Cordia dichotoma (*C. dichotoma*) leaves were examined for their anticancer activity by Rahman *et al.* [63]. The medicinal plant *C. dichotoma,* commonly named as *Boraginaceae* is is utilized for the treatment of different ailments in India. Leaves of *C. dichotoma* were used to treat the diseases such as demulcent, astringent, diuretic, antidiabetic, expectorant and anthelmintic. Leaves of *C. dichotoma* consist of flavonoids, phenolics and carotenoids showed good anticancer and antioxidant activities. Thus, investigators have aimed to explore the potential antiproliferative and apoptosis properties of methanolic extract of leaves of *C. dichotoma* (MECD) on human prostate carcinoma cell line. Along with the anticancer activity, total flavonoid content and also antioxidant activity were explored. *Soymida fembrifuga* (Roxb.) A. Juss. *Tinospora cordifolia* (Willd.) Miers., *Lavandula bipinnata* (L.) O. Ktze. and *Helicteres isora L.,* plants were selected for the study of anticancer property. These plants were dried and their extracts were obtained using hexane, ethanol and water as solvents. Human cancer cell lines HeLa−B75, HL−60, HEP−3B, PN−15 and normal liver cell lines were utilized in this study. With minute modification, MTT assay procedure was used to perform cytotoxicity assay and the percent cytotoxicity was computed. DMSO was used to dissolve MECD and absorbance of sample in each well of the plate was recorded at 540 nm by microplate Elisa reader. The well containing MTT without MECD was treated as control. Concentration lethal to 50% of the cancer cells (IC_{50}) was evaluated and morphology of cells was studied using inverted phase contrast microscopy. To evaluate the anticancer activity of plant extract, MTT assay was performed to study the cytotoxicity of PC3 cells. Process of induction of apoptosis was analyzed by DAPI (4’,6-diamidino-2-phenylindole) staining and level of intracellular reactive oxygen species (ROS) activity was scrutinized by 2,'7'-dichlorofluorescin diacetate (DCFH-DA) staining method. Anticancer effect of MECD sample against prostate carcinoma (PC3) cell line was examined by MTT assay. It suggested the significant changes in morphological shapes of the cells and these were noted to be dose-dependent mode. From the photomicrographs, it was evident that the shape of cells was changed to round along with detachment of cells from the surfaces in treated groups of cells. At higher concentrations of the sample, the investigators have observed the substantial death of cells. So, cell death was verified by experiments of cellular shrinkage, surface detachment and deformation of cells. The value of IC_{50} for the MECD extract was noted to be 74.5 mg/mL and the results of fluorescence DAPI (4',6-diamidino-2-phenylindole) staining test confirmed the nuclear apoptosis of cancer cells that was induced by MECD. Photomicrographs obtained by fluorescence DAPI staining exhibited apoptosis which included the condensed and fragmented nuclei in PC3 cells. Concurrently, results of DCFH-DA (2',7' -dichlorodihydrofluorescin diacetate) staining on PC3 cells indicated the level of ROS activity within the cellular premises which were persuaded by MECD extract. This prominent activity was confirmed by the fluorescence photomicrographs of stained PC3 cells and from the graph of percent dichlorofluorescein (DCF)-fluorescence *versus* concentration of MECD. Increased level of ROS activity in PC3 cell lines assisted the apoptosis over a number of pathways. Analysis of phytochemical compounds in MECD suggested the presence of alkaloid, saponins, steroid, carbohydrate, flavonoids, phenolics and cardiac glycosides. All these positive outcomes suggested that *C. dichotoma* could be a potent anticancer or a cancer chemopreventive agent.

Heliawati and coworkers worked on the extraction, isolation of active compound and biological activity of gewang seed extract [64]. The investigators have utilized *Corypha utan* Lamk that is used as fish poison in Timor Island (Indonesia) to isolate the anticancer compound. Murine leukemia P-388 cell lines were taken for antiproliferative study. Anticancer activity was performed by MTT assay using antonin E as positive control against the murine leukemia P-388 cell lines. Phosphate buffer solution of pH 7.30-7.65 was used to prepare the different concentrations of sample excluding control. Optical density was recorded at 540 nm by microplate reader. So, extrapolation of absorption line against different concentrations of sample resulted in IC_{50} value. Results drawn from UV-visible, Fourier transform infrared spectroscopy (FTIR) and ^{1}H NMR and ^{13}C NMR spectral studies confirmed that the isolated compound was piceatannol. Results of cytotoxicity activity test exhibited robust antiproliferative activity with IC_{50} value of 1.56 ppm. This suggested that piceatannol was active and could be used as an anticancer agent.

Five different vinca alkaloids were explored for their antiproliferative actions. The investigators of this study also examined alteration of spindle organization, blockage of mitosis and depolymerization of microtubules by vinca alkaloids [65]. Structure activity approach was used to investigate the suppressing ability of cell proliferation. Vinca alkaloids are well known effective inhibitors of cell propagation and are extensively used in the treatment of various cancers. Vinca alkaloids are largely used in cancer chemotherapy due to their tubulin binding nature thereby suppressing the multiplication of tubulin into microtubules. In specific, vinca alkaloids function as inhibiting agents and modify the activities of spindle microtubules and so results in proper function of chromosomes. Vincristine, vinblastine, vindesine, vinepidine and vinrosidine are used to prepare samples and were tested for antiproliferative activity. HeLa cancer cell line was taken and concentration-dependent inhibition of HeLa cell was quantified. Results showed that vinblastine exhibited greater inhibition with $K_{i,prol}$ value of 0.45 nM. The most weak inhibition potency was showed by vinrosidine with $K_{i,prol}$ value of 2200 nM. Antitubulin immunofluorescence microscopy was used to investigate the association and distribution of cells in control sample and drug treated sample. 4,'6-diamidino-2-phenylindole (DAPI) staining method was used to examine the organization and distribution. This suggested that cells were accumulated at metaphase stage. The data obtained from this investigation confirmed that cell cycle was inhibited at the metaphase stage of mitotic process. This inhibition of mitotic spindle has occurred at very low and operative concentrations of vinca alkaloids. Very little or no characteristic disruption was noticed in the spindle accretion or else same observation was made in microtubule depolymerization. As a result, the present study adds very excellent chemotherapeutic agent to the existing list of anticancer drugs and could be used in chemotherapy.

Euphorbia tirucalli (*E. tirucalli*), a traditional plant that belongs to *Euphorbiaceae,* is used for the ailments like asthma, cancer, syphilis, skin diseases, colic, intestinal parasites and leprosy [66]. This plant parts partly consist of some phenolics and terpenes, due to which it possess good and natural antioxidant properties. Latex of this plant is used for the treatment of cancer in traditional method. Extracts of leaf and/or stem of this plant possess powerful antioxidant properties which are crucial for opposing cellular oxidative stress. Increased level of phenolic content makes the plant extract to exhibit excellent antioxidant property. The present study used water for the extraction of sample because water is safe, eco-friendly, easily available and inexpensive compared to organic solvents. Since, methanol is also safe solvent, investigators of this study have also extracted plant content using it. Four different antioxidant assays were performed to compare the aqueous and methanolic extract for their total phytochemical actions and antioxidant ability. Response surface methodology (RSM) technique was used to optimize the aqueous extraction process and influence of extraction time, ratio of sample and solvent and temperature was investigated. The investigators have also concentrated on the antiproliferative activity of extract for which pancreatic cancer cells were used to test the samples. In order to get more potent agent from the *Euphorbia tirucalli*, plant extract was tested for all possible chemical analysis and total phenolic content (by Folin-Ciocalteu assay), total flavonoid content (modified aluminum chloride assay method) and total proanthocyanidin content (by vanillin-HCl method) was analyzed. Pancreatic cell viability was tested using human pancreatic cancer cell line-Mia-PaCa2 which is American Type Culture Collection (ATCC). These cell lines were cultured by means of Dulbecco's Modified Eagle's Medium (DMEM). Dojindo Cell Counting Kit-8 was used to determine the cell viability upon the addition of extract sample. Methanolic and aqueous extract sample of concentrations of 200, 100, 50, 25, 12.5 and 6.25 μg/mL were added to cells in well plate. Before determining cell viability, absorbance was noted at 450 nm. Results of cell viability analysis revealed that both methanolic and aqueous extracts possessed identical activity (at 50 μg/mL) of ~50% viability of cells. Toxicity of *E. tirucalli* was also tested which was dependent on concentration. Viability of cells was decreased with rise in the dose of plant extract. At the same time, all these findings suggested that ethanolic extract exhibited better activity in decreasing cell feasibility at 25 μg/mL when compared to that by aqueous extract. The experimental results demonstrated that *E. tirucalli* has good antiproliferative action and excellent antioxidant property.

Origanum include 23 species which is generally used for food and pharmaceutical industries. This is also utilized as folklore medicine for problems like indigestion, headache, muscle pains, diarrhea, rheumatism, asthma as herbal tea, *etc* [67]. Oil extracted from this plant is used as a flavoring agent in various foods, for example soups, sauces, fish, meat, canned foods and bitters. This genus plant exhibited good antioxidant, antiulceroge, antimicrobial, antiviral, antinociceptive, antitumor and antifungal properties. *Origanum rotundifolium* (*O. rotundifolium*) is a plant of genus called *Origanum* which is used by Erenler *et al.* to isolate phytochemicals and investigated the antioxidant and antiproliferative protperties. This genus plant consisted of diterpenes, flavonoids, steroids, monoterpenes, hydroquinone, hydroquinone monomethyl ether, flavone, glycosides *etc*. In order to determine the antiproliferative ability of plant extract, cell lines C6, HT29, HeLa and Vero were used. Dulbecco's modified eagle's medium was employed to culture these cell lines to which fetal bovine serum (FBS) and PenStep solution (ATCC, American Type Culture Collection) was added. For BrdU cell proliferation, enzyme linked immune solvent assay (ELISA) kit was used to test the cell proliferation against different cell lines. Half inhibitory concentration (IC_{50}) of the isolated moieties of extract and control sample was calculated and % inhibition was evaluated using the formula given below:

$$\% \text{ Inhibition} = [(A_{sample} - A_{control})/A_{control}] \text{ X } 100$$

where A_{sample} is the absorbance of the compound and $A_{control}$ is the absorbance of DMSO. For lactate dehydrogenase (LDH), cytotoxicity detection Kit (Roche, USA) was employed to test the cytotoxicity of isolated compounds and standard sample. For LDH assay C6, HT29, HeLa and Vero cells were utilized and its assay was performed by microplate reader by assessing the absorbance at 492-630 nm. Using *O. rotundifolium* plant extract the investigators of present study have isolated compounds called apigenin, rosmarinic acid, ferulic acid, vitexin, caprolactam and globoidnan A (shown in Figure 9) which are shown below:

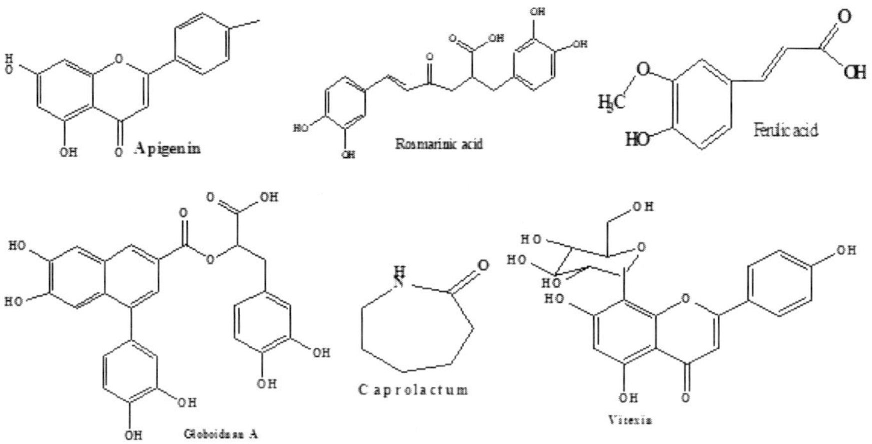

Figure 9. Chemical structure of isolated compounds.

Structures of isolated compounds were elucidated by spectroscopic techniques like one-dimensional (1D) NMR, liquid chromatography/time-of-flight/mass spectrometry (LC/TOF/MS) and two-dimensional (2D) NMR. Compared to all other isolated compounds, vitexin possessed highest activity towards C6 cells lines but for apigenin and caprolactum no significant effect was noticed. Various concentrations of extracted compounds were analyzed towards HeLa cell lines for human cervix carcinoma. Vitexin and ferulic acid exhibited the significant activity against HeLa cell lines compared to standard and other compounds. Rosmarinic acid and globoidnan A possessed moderate activity which might be due to the synergic effect while apigenin did not show the considerable action. Other compounds except apigenin exhibited good antiproliferative activity against HT29-human colon carcinoma cell lines. In addition to anticancer activity, extracted compounds also revealed good antioxidant property. All the isolated compounds have potent natural antioxidant property and could be used in pharmaceuticals.

Melastoma malabathricum (*M. malabathricum*) belongs to the family called *Melastomataceae* [68]. It is taken as testing sample in this study since it possesses anticancer activity. This plant was utilized as traditional medicine in Malays for the treatment of a number of ailments (reddened cuts, blood loss, pox marks, hemorrhoids and diarrhea). Literature survey has revealed the extract of *M. malabathricum* leaves in different solvents like ethanol, chloroform and water. These extracts exhibited different activities. Ethanolic extract possessed antinociceptive activity at both the peripheral and central levels which activated opioid receptors. Plant contained phytochemicals like β-sitosterol, sitosterol-3-*O*-β-D-glucopyranoside, quercetin, rutin and α-amyrin. Literature study has also disclosed that different extracts of the plant also showed antioxidant and cytotoxic activities. In this study, the investigators have aimed primarily to study the antiproliferative activity (*in vitro*). In addition, DPPH radical scavenging and superoxide scavenging assays were carried out. *In vitro* antiproliferative activity was evaluated against different cell lines. These are 3T3 for normal mouse fibroblast, HeLa- for human cervical adenocarcinoma, Caov-3- for human ovarian adenocarcinoma, MCF-7- for estrogen-dependent human breast adenocarcinoma, HL-60-for acute promyelocytic leukemia, CEM-SS- for T-lymphoblastic leukemia and MDA-MB-231- for human breast carcinoma. All cell lines were screened with three different extracts of plant (methanol, aqueous and chloroform). The data revealed the antiproliferative activity of *M. malabathricum* plant. Antioxidant property and radical scavenging actions of plant extract also contributed to the anticancer activity of the plant directly or indirectly. Various flavonoids present in the chloroform, aqueous, and methanol extracts showed encouraging kinase inhibition activity. Methanolic extract included saponins which exhibited apoptotic mechanism by permeabilization of the sheaths of mitochondria. In addition to this, saponins also caused cell death. Leave extract of *M. malabathricum* unveiled better antiproliferative activity against various cancer cell lines.

8.2. Antidiabetic Properties of Plants

Merremia tridentata (L.) Hall. f. (*M. tridentata*) is a plant of a family called *Convolvulaceae* [69]. It is also commonly known as Mudiarkunthal, Savulikodi, Thrippan Pullu in Tamil and Prasarini and has medicinal importance. This plant is used as folklore medicine to treat rheumatism, swelling, piles, wound curing, inflammation, arthritic and also for urinary problems. *M. tridentata* consist of flavanoids, luteolin, diosmetin, hygrins, nicotine and other flavanoids like ergosine alkaloids and 7-*O*-β-D-glucosides. The phenolic compounds of plant parts were found to have good antidiabetic property. Antidiabetic effect of aqueous extract of root of this plant was tested in rats of different conditions. For this normal, glucose loaded hyperglycemic and diabetic rat that was induced by streptozotocin (STZ) was used. This plant is also used in treating the rheumatism, swellings, piles and urinary disorders. Some studies illustrated the strong wound healing and anti-inflammatory actions of *M. tridentata.* Glucose in serum was evaluated using glucose estimation kit by glucose oxidase (GOD)-peroxidase (POD) method. Along with this serum insulin, serum triglycerides and serum total cholesterol were estimated by spectrophotometric method. Glycogen content in liver and skeletal muscle and *in vivo* lipid peroxidation in pancreatic tissue were also estimated by different reported methods. Effect of root extract on normoglycemic rats was found to be dose-dependent. Animals were treated with 50, 100 and 150 mg/kg sample and observed reduction in blood glucose level. Results of analysis on diabetic rat that was induced by streptozotocin (STZ) exhibited significant decrease in the insulin of blood. This study investigated hypoglycemic actions of *M. tridentata* root aqueous extract (MTRAE) in normal rats, glucose-loaded hyperglycemic rats and diabetic rats induced by streptozotocin. Increase in the level of insulin in animals induced by MTRAE indicated the efficiency of the extract in influencing the pancreatic secretion insulin by β-cells of islets of langerhans. A standard hypoglycemic drug, glibenclamide was used to compare the hyperglycemic actions of MTRAE. Before treatment of MTRAE, reduction was observed equally in muscle and hepatic glycogen. But, on treatment with 100 and 150 mg/kg of MTRAE for muscle and liver for some days revealed the drastic raise in the level of glycogen. This suggested the repair of defective storage of the glycogen by extract in the diabetic condition. In addition to this, MTRAE also cut down the level of serum triglycerides and total cholesterol diabetic rats treated by streptozotocin. MTRAE could change the deformity of total lipid level of the blood. Antioxidant actions of flavonoids helped to attenuate the increased lipid peroxidation which was induced by MTRAE. It was evident that the MTRAE has advantages like reduction of blood glucose and lipid. However, no negative effect was observed on normal rats.

Melastoma malabathricum (*M. malabathricum*) is a small shrub mainly found in cleared land, westeland, Asia and other parts of world [70]. *M. malabathricum* fall under the family called Melastomataceae which includes more than 4000 species of plants. In traditional medicinal therapy, many parts of this plant are utilized for treating common ailments. Roots and leaves of this plant are used to treat post-nasal care, wound, blemishes of small pox infection, dysentery, diarrhea and stomach ulcers, *etc.* This plant possesses antioxidant, antiinflammatory, antinociceptive, antipyretic, antifungal, antibacterial and antidiabetic activities. *n*-hexane, chloroform and methanol extracts were prepared for further studies. Human breast cancer cell lines, MCF-7 were used for the *in vitro* cytotoxicity test and determination of cell viability. Methylene blue (MB) staining method was used since it stains only the feasible cells. Dose-response curve was obtained from non-linear regression analysis and cytotoxicity was evaluated by the same curve. Results of cytotoxicity test revealed that methanol extract of leaf and flower illustrated significant inhibition (81.23 and 77.97%, respectively for leaf and flower) of MCF-7 cells compared to that of extract of stem. Likewise results of dose-dependent test indicated that all the extracts showed increased activity upon treatment of long term. *M. malabathricum* showed good anticancer activity against MCF-7 cell lines with IC_{50} value less than 25 μg/mL. So, these findings highlighted the potential anticancer property of the leaf and flower extract of the sample.

Garlic (*Allium sativum* L.) is mainly utilized for medicinal use. Garlic cloves contain allinase enzyme that helps to produce allicin from alliin [71]. Allicin is the active compound present in garlic. Likewise turmeric (*Curcuma longa*) is also a well-known spice and is utilized as a medicinal plant in some Asian countries including India. Curcuma species contains active component called curcuminoids which exhibit various biological properties. Among curcuminoids, curcumin is one dynamic element which is responsible for several pharmacological effects. Reduction of total blood cholesterol and decrease in level of glucose, *etc*., are the significant pharmacological properties showed by curcuma. A number of plants have been used for medicinal purposes. Among them, *Curcuma longa* and *Allium sativum* L. also unveil hypoglycemic action and hence are used in treating diabetes. The investigators have studied the ability and safety of curcuma in type 2 diabetes with glibenclamide in the presence and absence of dyslipidemia. Several new effective antidiabetic agents and antihyperglycemic agents have been developed. Preparation of insulin from different sources also been innovated robustly. From the preclinical and clinical trials, it was found and confirmed that the combination of garlic and turmeric extract portrays exhibited good antidiabetic activity. In addition, trial of this extract on animal also showed synergistic effect that is not found with the use of an individual extract. For this study, the investigators have tried the prepared extract on male/female patients (aged more than 35 years) suffering from type 2 diabetes mellitus. The samples of patients have been tested for random blood glucose level (≥200 mg/dL), fasting blood glucose level (≥126 mg/dL) and with/without dyslipidemia. The samples of all the patients were analyzed for total blood glucose, total lipid and also screed for other hematological assays. No adverse effect was noticed or reported upon the treatment of prepared extract and the extract was acted equally to glibenclamide. At the end, prepared extract decreased the blood glucose and lipid levels within well tolerance in the body.

Literature survey revealed that plants/plant parts such as *Geigeria alata* (*G. alata*), *Acacia nilotica, Balanites aegyptiaca, Guiera senegalensis, Hyphaene thebaica* and *Trigonella foenum-graecum* possessed hyperglycemic activity and was used mainly in western Sudan [72]. *Tinospora cordifolia, Mitragyna inremis* (Wild) O. Kundze (*M. inremis*) and *Nauclea latifolia* (*N. latifolia*) are well known for their antidiabetic actions. Present study aimed to examine the antidiabetic effect of the aqueous extract of plants like *M. inremis, N. latifolia, R. nilotica, T. bakis* and *S. hermonthica*. Toxicity test of selected plant extracts was analyzed by carrying out tests on animals. No side effect/toxic effect was observed up to higher dose of extract. Results of test on oral glucose tolerance were examined for normal control rats; streptozocin (STZ) induced diabetic rats (control) and diabetic rats treated with glibenclamide. Blood glucose level was reduced drastically in diabetic rats treated with aqueous extracts of *T. bakis, N. latifolia* and *R. nilotica* ($p < 0.05$). However, extracts of *S. hermonthica* and *M. inremis* did not exhibit significant decrease in the blood glucose. Changes in high-density lipoprotein cholesterol (HDL-C) and low-density lipoprotein cholesterol (LDL-C) levels were noticed. Influence of plants extracts on diabetic liver and kidney function markers, changes in the level of creatinine, urea and blood urea nitrogen, total triglycerides levels, fasting blood glucose and total cholesterol levels was examined in detail. Renal dysfunction/disturbance in metabolism led to increase in the levels of renal function parameters in diabetic rats. *M. inremis* significantly reduced urea and blood urea nitrogen level while *T. bakis* and *R. nilotica* decreased ($p < 0.05$) the level of creatinine. *N. latifolia* effectively influenced the level of blood urea nitrogen. The present study illustrated well the efficiency of some plants of western Sudan in treating the diabetic and related abnormalities of body.

Present study investigates antidiabetic activity of different plants namely *Brassica juncea* (*B. juncea*), *Combretum micranthum* (*C. micranthum*), *Elephantopus scaber* (*E. scaber*), *Gymnema sylvestre* (*G. sylvestre*), *Liriope spicata* (*L. spicata*), *Parinari excelsa* (*P. excelsa*), *Ricinus communis* (*R. communis*), *Sarcopoterium spinosum* (*S. spinosum*),

Smallanthus sonchifolius (*S. sonchifolius*), *Swertia punicea* (*S. punicea*), and *Vernonia anthelmintica* (*V. anthelmintica*) [73]. *B. juncea* belongs to family, *Cruciferae* which is used in traditional medicinal therapy. Seed extract of *B. juncea* in aqueous form possess effective hypoglycemic actions. Antidiabetic effect of aqueous extract was analyzed on STZ induced diabetic rats. Results of this test revealed good hypoglycemic activity at 250, 350, 450 mg/kg doses. *Eugenia jambolana* (*E. jambolana*) is well known in the name of Jamun or Indian blackberry. This plant is being used in Indian medicinal therapy for diabetic problem. Results of both experimental and clinical test unraveled hypoglycemic effect of the extract of *E. jambolana*. Likewise, *Coccina grandis* (*C. grandis*) leaves possessed hypoglycemic activity. Alcoholic extracts of *C. grandis* leaves (dose limit of 600 mg/kg) noteworthy antidiabetic effect on normal fasted rats. Leaves extract injected in rats significantly reduced blood glucose level. Methanolic extract of *Albizia odoratissima* bark was tested for hypoglycemic effect. The alloxan dosage of 250 and 500 mg/kg was injected in to the induced diabetic mice. As a result, considerable reduction in the levels of serum cholesterol, triglycerides, alkaline phosphatase and total proteins in alloxan induced mice was noticed. Anti-diabetic action of the leaf extract of the plant called *Axonopus compressus* (*A. compressus*) was investigated. Leave extract obtained from methanol solvent was used and injected in to alloxan induced rats. A. compressus showed excellent decrement in the blood glucose levels at doses of 250, 500 and 1000 mg/kg, compared to that in the control rat. It revealed the significant antidiabetic actions of *A. compressus*. Finally, this study unraveled antidiabetic efficacy of various medicinal plants.

Present study examines the influence of active components present in leaves of *Leptadenia reticulate (L. reticulate)* on blood glucose. Ethanolic extract of leaves of *L. reticulate* (ETLR) was used for the isolation of compounds by chromatographic techniques [74]. Effect of isolated fraction of ETLR and metformin were tested by administering orally. So, pure compound was isolated from fractions possessing higher antidiabetic activity by column chromatography (CC). Pure compound obtained was named as LR-1 (trivial name). A fraction of ETLR was effective in lowering the level of fasting blood glucose (FBG) considerably with $p < 0.05$ mainly in STZ induced diabetic rats. Various solvent systems were used to carry out column chromatographic analysis for the fraction of ETLR. Spectral analysis (FTIR, ^{13}C-NMR, ^{1}H-NMR and mass spectra) was performed to confirm the nature of LR-1 as phenolic compound (flavonoids). The fraction called "D" that was isolated from ETLR exhibited robust antidiabetic activity in comparison to a standard called metformin. The exact mechanism of action of the fraction, LR-1 was not yet understood and it could be subjected to further investigation.

Medicinal plants like *Aporosa lindleyana* Baill, *Gentiana olivieri* griseb, *Bauhinia forficata koeingii*, *Lactuca indica* L., *Eugenia jambolana* L., *Momordica charantia* L., *Mucuna pruriens* Bak., Cogent db, *Myrtus communis* L., *Rhizoma Polygonati Odorati*, *Tinospora cordifolia* W., and *Terminalia pallida* Brand showed good antidiabetic activity [75]. Most of these are excellent hypoglycemic and anti-hyperglycemic agents. It is well known that compared to other plants, *Pterocarpus marsupium* Roxb., *Momordica charantia* L., and *Trigonella foenum* greacum L. are effective agents to treat type 2 diabetes. *Aporosa lindleyana* Baillplant of Euphorbiaceae family was tested for the antihyperglycemic activity by preparing the aqueous and alcoholic extracts. *Aporosa lindleyana* Baill considerably decreased the blood glucose in alloxan-induced diabetic rats (3069/3.37 to 1609/2.46 and 3289/4.15 to 1529/3.86 mg%). I) Using the standard, tolbutamide which is an oral hypoglycemic agent, antihyperglycemic actions of plant sample was equated. II) It was found that extracts of *Momordica charantia* (*M. charantia*) L., *Eugenia jambolana* (*E. jambolana*) L., *Tinospora cordifolia* (*T. cordifolia*) W., and *Mucuna pruriens* (*M. pruriens*) Bak., significantly reduced the blood glucose level in STZ-induced diabetic rats. So, extracts of all these plants efficiently inhibited the polyuria condition mainly in diabetic controlled rats. In addition, the investigators observed significant reduction in urine albumin levels upon treatment with prepared extract of plants. Extract of *E. jambolana* and *M. charantia* showed effective actions towards renal hypertrophy and completely prevented. III) *Pterocarpus marsupium* (*P. marsupium*) Roxb., *Trigonella foenum-graecum* L. (*T. foenum-graecum*) and *Ocimum sanctum* (*O. sanctum*) L. plant parts were selected to investigate their hypoglycemic effect. Aqueous bark extract of *P. marsupium* and alcoholic extract for seed of *T. foenum-graecum* and leaves of *O. sanctum* were prepared and used for further study. Three extracts were tested for normal and alloxan-induced diabetic rats. Results of analysis indicated that the aqueous extract of *P. marsupium* ($p < 0.001$) decreased blood sugar levels suggestively from 72.32 ± 5.62 to 61.35 ± 1.2 mg/kg/BW) after the immediate administration of prepared extract. The investigators also noticed lowering of blood glucose in alloxan induced diabetic mice (from 202.91 ± 5.44 to 85.22 ± 11.28 mg/kg/BW) after 21 days of the oral administration. Further, it was found that blood glucose level was reduced with alcoholic extract of *T. foenum-graecum* ($p < 0.001$) and also in *O. sanctum* ($p < 0.001$). IV). Rhizoma *Polygonati Odorati* (R. *Polygonati Odorati*), found in the family Liliaceae, exhibited its effect on glucose/carbohydrate metabolism mainly in diabetic animals *via* different roots. For example, it may suppress the activity of α-glucosidase and helps to improve the glucose and triglyceride metabolic pathway. Extract of R. *Polygonati Odorati* declined the level of both hyperglycemia and hypertriglyceridemia in diabetic rats with hyperlipemia. V) *Terminalia pallida* Brandis (*T. brandis*) belongs to *Combretaceae* family and is one important plant which possesses antidiabetic activity. Then, ethanolic extract of *T. brandis* was orally administered to alloxan-induced diabetic rats. When a dosage of 0.5g/kg body weight (bw) of ethanolic extract was injected, the investigators have observed excellent antihyperglycemic activity while no significant result of hypoglycemic activity was observed in normal rats. Likewise, *Tinospora cordifolia* (*T. cordifolia*) was investigated for the hypolipidemic effect. Roots of this plant were used as sample material to test its efficacy to decrease the body cholesterol. Results obtained upon the administration of root extract for 45 days unraveled the considerable decrease in cholesterol, free fatty acids and phospholipids content in both serum and tissue. Efficiency of root extract was compared to that of standard pharmaceutical agent, glibenclamide. Results of this study suggested that the administration of *T. cordifolia* W. roots was better at 2.5 and 5.0 g/kg body weight (bw) when compared to the effect of glibenclamide.

Gymnema sylvestre (*G. sylvestre*) is a climbing plant found mainly in tropical forest of some parts of India [76]. It has common name called gurmar, since its leaves have the capacity to neutralize the taste sense for sugar. Alcoholic extract of leaves of this plant was taken as sample material. Prepared extract was tested on normal and anterior pituitary injected hyperglycemic mice (at a dose of 100 mg/kg). Alcoholic extract of leaves was used for the isolation of active components and is named as GS4. Treatment of a water soluble extract GS4 obtained from the leaves of *Gymnema sylvestre* to STZ induced rats resulted in increased level of beta cells in pancreas. Along with that, GS4 also inhibited the level of blood sugar in the body by suppressing the glucose uptake action from the intestine. So, it indicated that the leave extract of *G. sylvestre* plant is capable of reducing the blood glucose level. *Ficus benga/ensis* is commonly called as Banyan tree in English, which is worshiped in India. The aerial roots and leaves of this plant are well known for the treatment of ulcers. It produces juice which is milky in nature and is used to cure the pain and skin damages, cuts and also for the rheumatism. Aerial roots of *F. benga* are useful to treat syphilis, dysentery, gonorrhea and liver inflammation. From the literature survey, it was found that, compared to other parts of this plant, bark has very good antidiabetic activity. To investigate the hypoglycemic effect of bark, the extract of bark was prepared and treated for the alloxan-induced diabetic animals like rabbits, rats and humans. Aqueous extract of bark was isolated from the *F. benga.* It showed effective antidiabetic property at a very low dose of 10 mg/kg, body weight/day. *Momordica charantia* (*M. charantia*) is common vegetable plant; its fruits are widely used. It has common name called bitter gourds in English and Karela in Hindi. In India *M. charantia*is extensively used for the treatment of diabetes mellitus. Fruits of *M. charantia* have the capacity to reduce the blood sugar level and also help in improving the tolerance of glucose in the body. Extract of fruit exhibited good effect when treated it on STZ-induced diabetic mice. The alcoholic extract of fruit possessed a considerable decrease in the fasting blood sugar in alloxan-induced rabbits. The polypeptide that was isolated from *M. charantia* was found to be similar to the bovine insulin in its action on diabetes mellitus. Under the clinical trials, isolated polypeptide showed 45% reduction in the blood glucose level. All these results clearly suggested that *M. charantia* and its fruit was effective to treat the diabetic condition.

CONCLUSION

The current chapter revealed the role of medicinal plants in providing the effective antidiabetic and anticancer agents to the world. Utilization of medicinal plants for the prevention and treatment of chronic diseases is a great challenge in the modern medicinal therapy. Practice of herbal medicinal therapy has created a new world in the medicinal field. We have reviewed a number of whole plants/plant parts that play a proficient role in the treatment of cancer and diabetis mellitus. We have discussed the preparation and utilization of a huge number of active contents of plants that are capable of curing different types of cancers effectively. Scientific community has developed new therapies and drugs against death causing diseases like cancer and diabetes. Success in realizing certain bioactive phytochemicals has resulted in the creation of a number of staple drugs and development of efficient technologies for the treatment of several life threatening health problems.

REFERENCES

[1] Dillard CJ, German JB. Phytochemicals: neutraceuticals and human health. *Journal of Science of Food and Agriculture* 80(12), 1744-1756, 2000.

[2] Ramakrishna S, Ramana KV, Mihira V, Kumar BP. Evaluation of anti-inflammatory and analgesic activities of *Solanum trilobatum* Linn. roots. *Res J Pharm Biol Chem Sci* 2(1), 701-705, 2011.

[3] https:// www. mentalhelp. net/ articles/ overview- introduction- to-cancer/.

[4] https:// www.mayoclinic.org/ diseases-conditions/ cancer/ symptoms-causes/syc-20370588.

[5] https://en.wikipedia.org/wiki/Causesofcancer.

[6] https://www.medicinenet.com/cancer/article.htm.

[7] https://www.emedicinehealth.com/cancer_symptoms/article_em.htm #what_are_18_signs_and_symptoms_of_cancer.

[8] https://www.cancer.gov/about-cancer/treatment/types.

[9] https://en.wikipedia.org/wiki/Treatment_of_cancer.

[10] https://www.cancer.gov/about-cancer/treatment/side-effects.

[11] https://www.cancer.org/treatment/treatments-and-side-effects/treatment-types/targeted-therapy/side-effects.html.

[12] Wang H, Khor TO, Shu L, Su Z, Fuentes F, Lee JH, Kong ANT. Plants against cancer: A review on natural phytochemicals in preventing and treating cancers and their druggability. *Anticancer Agents Med Chem* 12(10), 1281–1305, 2012.

[13] http://chemoth.com/types/vincaalkaloids.

[14] https://en.wikipedia.org/wiki/Vinca_alkaloid.

[15] Moudi M, Go R, Yien CY, Nazre M. Vinca alkaloids. *Int J Prev Med* 4(11), 1231-1235, 2013.

[16] Sultana N, Lee NH, Antielastase and free radical scavenging activities of compounds from stems of *Cornus kousa. Phytotherapy Res* 21(12), 117-1176, 2007.

[17] Gangan VD, Pradhan P, Sipahimalani AT. Phytoecdysones from *Tinospora cordifolia*: Structural elucidation of ecdysterone and makisterone A by 2D NMR spectroscopy. *Indian J Chem* 36(B), 787-792, 1997.

[18] Chopra RN, Chopra LC, Handa KD, Kapur LD. *Indigenous Drugs of India*. 2nd edition, pp. 426-428, 1956. Calcutta. Dhar VN. and Sons, India.

[19] https://www.healthline.com/health/diabetes/types-of-diabetes.

[20] https://www.webmd.com/diabetes/guide/types-of-diabetes-mellitus#1.

[21] Kooti W, Farokhipour M, Asadzadeh Z, Ashtary-Larky D, Asadi-Samani M. The role of medicinal plants in the treatment of diabetes: a systematic review. *Electron Physician* 8(1), 1832-1842, 2016.

[22] Ocvirk S, Kistler M, Khan S, Talukder SH, Hauner H. Traditional medicinal plants used for the treatment of diabetes in rural and urban areas of Dhaka, Bangladesh–an ethnobotanical survey. *Journal of Ethnobiology and Ethnomedicine* 9:43, 2013. http://www.ethnobiomed.com/content/9/1/43.

[23] Kumar R, Patel DK, Prasad SK, Laloo D, Krishnamurthy S, Hemalatha S. Type 2 antidiabetic activity of bergenin from the roots of *Caesalpinia digyna* Rottler. *Fitoterpia* 83(2), 395-401, 2012.

[24] Ibeh BO, Ezeaja MI. Preliminary study of antidiabetic activity of the methanolic leaf extract of *Axonopus compressus* (*P. Beauv*) in alloxan-induced diabetic rats. *J Ethnopharmacol* 138(3), 713-716, 2011.

[25] Kumar D, Kumar S, kohli S, Arya R, Gupta J. Antidaibetic activity of methanolic bark extract of *Albizia odoratissima* Benth in alloxan-induced diabetic albino mice. *Asian Pac J Trop Med* 4(11), 900-903, 2011.

[26] Thirumalai T, Therasa VS, Elumalai EK, David E. Hypoglycemic effect of *Brassica juncea* (seeds) on streptozotocin induced diabetic male albino rat. *Asian Pac J Trop Biomed* 1(4), 323-325, 2011.

[27] Meliani N, Dib Mel A, Allali H, Tabti B. Hypoglycaemic effect of *Berberis vulgaris* L. in normal and streptozotocin induced diabetic rats. *Asian Pac J Trop Biomed*1(6), 468-471, 2011.

[28] Kumar R, Pate DK, Prasad SK, Sairam K, Hemalatha S. Antidiabetic activity of alcoholic leaves extract of *Alangium lamarckii* Thwaites on streptozotocin nicotinamide induced type 2 diabetic rats. *Asian Pac J Trop Med* 4(11), 904-909, 2011.

[29] Sefi M, Fetoui H, Lachkar N, Tahraoui A, Lyoussi B, Boudawara T, Zeghal N. *Centaurium erythrea* (Gentianaceae) leaf extract alleviates

streptozotocin-induced oxidative stress and β-cell damage in rat pancreas. *J Ethnopharmacol* 135(2), 243-250, 2011.

[30] Sancheti S, Sancheti S, Seo SY, Antidiabetic and anti-acetyl cholinesterase effects of ethyl acetate fraction of *Chaenomeles sinensis* (Thouin) Koehne fruits in streptozotocin induced diabetic rats. *Exp Toxicol Pathol* 65(1-2), 55-60, 2013.

[31] Ohadoma SC, Michael HU, Effects of co-administration of methanol leaf extract of *Catharanthus roseus* on the hypoglycemic activity of metformin and glibenclamide in rats. *Asian Pac J Trop Med* 4(6), 475-477, 2011.

[32] Eliza J, Diasy P, Ignacimuthu S, Duraipandiyan V. Antidiabetic and antilipidemic effect of eremanthin from *Costus speciosus* (Koen.) Sm., in STZ-induced diabetic rats. *Chem Biol Interact* 182(1), 67-72, 2009.

[33] Li S, Li J, Guan XL, Li J, Deng SP, Li LQ, Tang MT, Huang JG, Chen ZZ, Yang RY. Hypoglycemic effects and constituents of the barks of *Cyclocarya paliurus* and their inhibiting activities to glucosidase and glycogen phosphorylase. *Fitoterapia* 82(7), 1081-1085, 2011.

[34] Naskar S, Mazumder UK, Pramanik G, Gupta M, Kumar RB, Bala A, Islam A. Evaluation of antihyperglycemic activity of *Cocos nucifera* Linn. on streptozotocin induced type 2 diabetic rats. *J Ethnopharmacol* 138(3), 769-773, 2011.

[35] Patel DK, Kumar R, Prasad SK, Sairam K, Hemalatha S. Antidiabetic and *in vitro* antioxidant potential of *Hybanthus enneaspermus* (Linn) F. Muell in streptozotocin-induced diabetic rats. *Asian Pac J Trop Biomed* 1(4), 316-322, 2011.

[36] Hou SZ, Chen SX, Huang S, Jiang DX, Zhou CJ, Chen CQ, Liang YM, Lai XP. The hypoglycemic activity of *Lithocarpus polystachyus* Rehd. leaves in the experimental hyperglycemic rats. *J Ethnopharmacol* 138(1), 142- 149, 2011.

[37] Elberry AA, Harraz FM, Ghareib SA, Gabr SA, Nagy AA, Abdel-Sattar E. Methanolic extract of *Marrubium vulgare* ameliorates

hyperglycemia and dyslipidemia in streptozotocin-induced diabetic rats. *Int J Diabetes Mellitus* 3(1), 37-44, 2015.

[38] Patil R, Patil R, Ahirwar B, Ahirwar D. Isolation and characterization of anti-diabetic component (bioactivity-guided fractionation) from *Ocimum sanctum* L. (Lamiaceae) aerial part. *Asian Pac J Trop Med* 4(4), 278-282, 2011.

[39] Khan HB, Vinayagam KS, Sekar A, Palanivelu S, Panchanatham S. Antidiabetic and antioxidant effect of *Semecarpus anacardium* Linn. nut milk extract in a high-fat diet STZ-induced type 2 diabetic rat model. *J Diet Suppl* 9(1), 19-33, 2012; Khan HB, Vinayagam KS, Palanivelu S, Panchanatham S. Anti-diabetic effect of *Semecarpus anacardium* Linn nut milk extract in a high fat diet STZ-induced type 2 diabetic rat model. *Comp Clin Pathol* 21(6), 1395-1400, 2012.

[40] Sunil C, Ignacimuthu S, Agastian P. Antidiabetic effect of *Symplocos cochinchinensis* (Lour.) S. Moore. in type 2 diabetic rats. *J Ethnopharmacol* 134(2), 298-304, 2011.

[41] Ghoul JE, Ghanem-Boughanmi N, Ben-Attia M. Biochemical study on the protective effect of ethanolic extract of *Zygophyllum album* on streptozotocin-induced oxidative stress and toxicity in mice. *Biomedicine&Preventive Nutrition* 1(2), 79-83, 2011.

[42] Feshani AM, Kouhsari SM, Mohammadi S. *Vaccinium arctostaphylos*, a common herbal medicine in Iran: molecular and biochemical study of its antidiabetic effects on alloxan-diabetic Wistar rats. *J Ethnopharmacol* 133(1), 67-74, 2011.

[43] Bnouham M, Ziyyat A, Mekhfi H, Tehri A, Abdelkhaleg L. Medicinal plants with potential antidiabetic activity-A review of ten years of herbal medicine research (1990-2000). *International Journal of Diabetes and Metabolism* 14(1), 1-25, 2006.

[44] Chauhan A, Sharma PK, Srivastava Kumar PN, Dudhe R. Plants having potential antidiabetic activity: A review. Scholars Research Library. *Der Pharmacia Lettre* 2(3), 369-387, 2010.

[45] Nimenibo-Uadia R. Control of hyperlipidaemia, hypercholesterolaemia and hyperketonaemia by aqueous extract of

Dioscorea dumetorum tuber. *Tropical Journal of Pharmaceutical Research* 2(1), 183-189, 2003.

[46] Bhatia V, Kinja K, Bishnoi H, Savita S, Gnaneshwari D. Antidiabetic activity of the alcoholic extract of the arial part of *Boerhaavia diffusa* in rats. *Recent Research in Science and Technology* 3(7), 4-7, 2011.

[47] Adebayo J, Adesokan AA, Olatunji LA, Buoro DO, Soladoye AO. Effect of ethanolic extract of *Bougainvillea spectabilis* leaves on haematological and serum lipid variables in rats. *Biokemistri (Nigerian Society for Experimental Biology)* 17(1), 45-50, 2005.

[48] Muralikrishna KS, Latha KP, Shreedhara CS, Vaidya VP, Krupanidhi AM. Effect of *Bauhinia purpurea* Linn. on alloxan-induced diabetic rats and isolated frog's heart. *International Journal of Green Pharmacy* 2(2), 83-86, 2008.

[49] Kshirsagar RP, Darade SS, Takale V. Effect of *Alangium salvifolium* (Alangiaceae) on dexamethasone induced insulin resistance in rats. *J Pharm Res* 3(11), 2714-2716, 2010.

[50] Saxena A, Vikram NK. Role of selected Indian plants in management of type 2 diabetes: a review. *J Altern Complement Med* 10(2), 369-378, 2004.

[51] Ayodhya S, Kusum S, Anjali S. Hypoglycamic activity of different extracts of various herbal plants. *International Journal of Research in Ayurveda & Pharmacy* 1(1), 212-224, 2010.

[52] Wei LS, Wee W, Siong JY, Syamsumir DF. Characterization of anticancer, antimicrobial, antioxidant properties and chemical compositions of *Peperomia pellucida* leaf extract. *Acta Med Iran* 49(10), 670-674, 2011.

[53] Alaklabi A, Arif IA, Ahamed A, Kumar RS, Idhayadhulla A. Evaluation of antioxidant and anticancer activities of chemical constituents of the *Saururus chinensis* root extracts. *Saudi Journal of Biological Sciences* 25(7), 1387–1392, 2018.

[54] Mishra T, Arya RK, Meena S, Joshi P, Pal M, Meena B, Upreti DK, Rana TS, Dipak Datta D. Isolation, characterization and anticancer potential of cytotoxic triterpenes from *Betula utilis* bark. *PLoS One* 11(7): e0159430, 2016.

[55] Vemuri SK, Banala RR, Subbaiah GPV, Srivastava SK, Reddy AVG, Malarvili T. Anti-cancer potential of a mix of natural extracts of turmeric, ginger and garlic: A cell-based study. *Egyptian Journal of Basic and Applied Sciences* 4(4), 332-344, 2017.

[56] Yen GC, Chen CS, Chang WT, Wu MF, Cheng FT, Shiau DK, Hsu CL. Antioxidant activity and anticancer effect of ethanolic and aqueous extracts of the roots of *Ficus beecheyana* and their phenolic components. *J Food Drug Anal* 26(1), 182-192, 2018.

[57] Turan I, Demir S, Kilinc K, Burnaz NA, Yaman SO, Akbulut K, Mentese A, Aliyazicioglu Y, Deger O. Antiproliferative and apoptotic effect of *Morus nigra* extract on human prostate cancer cells. *Saudi Pharm J* 25(2), 241-248, 2017.

[58] Gavamukulya Y, Abou-Elella F, Wamunyokoli F, AEl-Shemy H. Phytochemical screening, anti-oxidant activity and *in vitro* anticancer potential of ethanolic and water leaves extracts of *Annona muricata* (Graviola). *Asian Pac J Trop Med* 7(Suppl 1), S355-S363, 2014.

[59] Balasubramanian K, Padma PR. Anticancer activity of *Zea mays* leaf extracts on oxidative stress-induced Hep2 cells. *J Acupunct Meridian Stud* 6(3), 149-58, 2013.

[60] Ghagane SC, Puranik SI, Kumbar VM, Nerli RB, Jalalpure SS, Hiremath MB, Neelagund S, Aladakatti R. *In vitro* antioxidant and anticancer activity of *Leea indica* leaf extracts on human prostate cancer cell lines. *Integr Med Res* 6(1), 79-87, 2017.

[61] Venugopal R, Liu RH. Phytochemicals in diets for breast cancer prevention: The importance of resveratrol and ursolic acid. *Food Science and Human Wellness* 1, 1–13, 2012.

[62] Raj GG, Varghese HS, Kotagiri S, Swamy BMV, Swamy A, Pathan RK. Anticancer studies of aqueous extract of roots and leaves of *Pandanus Odoratissimus* f. ferreus (Y. Kimura) Hatus; An *in vitro* approach. *Journal of Traditional and Complementary Medicine* 4(4), 279-284, 2014.

[63] Rahman MA, Siddiqui S, Akhtar J. Evaluation of anticancer activity of *Cordia dichotoma* leaves against a human prostate carcinoma cell

line, PC3. *Journal of Traditional and Complementary Medicine* 7(3), 315-321, 2017.

[64] Heliawati L, Kardinan A, Mayanti T, Tjokronegoro RA. Piceatannol: Anti-cancer compound from gewang seed extract. *Journal of Applied Pharmaceutical Science* 5(01), 110-113, 2015.

[65] Jordan MA, Thrower D, Wilson L. Mechanism of inhibition of cell proliferation by vinca alkaloids. *Cancer Res* 51(8), 2212-2222, 1991.

[66] Munro B, Vuong QV, Chalmers AC, Goldsmith CD, Bowyer MC, Scarlett CJ. Phytochemical, antioxidant and anti-cancer properties of *Euphorbia tirucalli* methanolic and aqueous extracts. *Antioxidants (Basel)* 4(4), 647-661, 2015.

[67] Erenler R, Meral B, Sen O, Elmastas M, Aydin A, Eminagaoglu O, Topcu G. Bioassay-guided isolation, identification of compounds from *Origanum rotundifolium* and investigation of their antiproliferative and antioxidant activities. *Pharm Biol* 55(1), 1646-1653, 2017.

[68] Zakaria ZA, Rofiee MS, Mohamed AM, Teh LK, Salleh MZ. *In vitro* antiproliferative and antioxidant activities and total phenolic contents of the extracts of *Melastoma malabathricum*leaves. *J Acupunct Meridian Stud* 4(4), 248-256, 2011.

[69] Arunachalam K, Parimelazhagan T. Antidiabetic activity of aqueous root extract of *Merremia tridentata* (L.) Hall. f. in streptozotocin-induced-diabetic rats. *Asian Pac J Trop Med* 5(3), 175-179, 2012.

[70] Roslen NA, Alewi NA, Ahamada H, Rasad MS. Cytotoxicity screening of *Melastoma malabathricum* extracts on human breast cancer cell lines *in vitro*. *Asian Pac J Trop Biomed* 4(7), 545-548, 2014.

[71] Sukandar EY, Sudjana P, Adnyana K, Setiawan AS, Yuniarni U. Recent study of turmeric in combination with garlic as antidiabetic agent. *Procedia Chemistry* 13, 44-56, 2014.

[72] Alamin MA, Yagi AI, Yagi SM. Evaluation of antidiabetic activity of plants used in Western Sudan. *Asian Pac J Trop Biomed* 5(5), 395-402, 2015.

[73] Arumugam G, Manjula P, Paari N. A review: Anti diabetic medicinal plants used for diabetes mellitus. *Journal of Acute Disease* 196-200, 2013. doi: 10.1016/S2221-6189(13)60126-2.

[74] Natarajan V, Dhas ASAG. Isolation and characterization of anti-diabetic compound from *Leptadenia reticulate* [w&a] leaf. *Integrative Obesity and Diabetes* 1(2), 36-40, 2015.

[75] Jung M, Park M, Lee HC, Kang YH, Kang ES, Kim SK. Antidiabetic agents from medicinal plants. *Curr Med Chem* 13(10), 1203-1218, 2006.

[76] Shukla R, Sharma SB, Puri D, Prabhu KM, Murthy PS. Medicinal plants for treatment of diabetes mellitus. *Indian Journal of Clinical Biochemistry* 15(Suppl 1), 169-177, 2000.

In: Natural Anti-Aging Plants …
Editor: Noboru Motohashi
ISBN: 978-1-53616-282-0

Chapter 3

THEOBROMA CACAO L.: A SOURCE OF FLAVONOIDS WITH IMPORTANT HEALTH RELATED EFFECTS

Carla Patricia Plazola-Jacinto[1,*], Marcela Hernández-Ortega[2,†] and Lourdes Valadez-Carmona[3,‡]

[1]Departamento de Ingeniería Bioquímica, Escuela Nacional de Ciencias Biológicas, Instituto Politécnico Nacional, México
[2]Facultad de Ciencias de la Salud, Universidad Anáhuac Norte México, Naucalpan de Juárez, Estado de México, México
[3]Centro de Investigación en Ciencias Biológicas Aplicadas, Universidad Autónoma del Estado de México, México

[*] Corresponding Author's E-mail: patricia.plazola@gmail.com.
[†] Corresponding Author's E-mail: marcelahdz17@yahoo.com.mx.
[‡] Corresponding Author's E-mail: lvc24@hotmail.com.

Abstract

Theobroma cacao is a plant used into chocolate manufacturing. Cacao and cacao-derived products are natural sources of bioactive compounds, these compounds are already known to have biological activities and health related effects. The main bioactive compounds found in cacao are polyphenols mostly flavonoids (**4**) such as ((-)-epicatechin (**1**), (+)-catechin (**2**), and oligomeric procyanidins (**3**)). Epidemiological studies highlight the association between cacao flavonoids (**4**) consumption and health effects, such as reduction of the risk of diabetes, affect the endothelial function, blood pressure and cholesterol level. Currently, studies are focused on cacao consumption and its relation with aging complications; the outcomes found so far, are a direct relation between cacao consumption and better life expectancy, and prevention or reduction of neurodegenerative diseases, which make flavonoids (**4**) a functional ingredients for pharmaceutical and cosmetic industries, to treat diverse diseases.

Keywords: flavonoids, cacao, life expectancy improvement, neurodegenerative diseases prevention

Abbreviations

(-)-epicatechin (**1**)
epicatechin (**1’**)
(+)-catechin (**2**)
catechin(s) (**2’**)
oligomeric procyanidins (**3**)
flavonoid(s) (**4**)
flavones (**5**)
flavonols (**6**)
flavan-3-ols (flavanols) (**7**)
isoflavones (**8**)
flavanones (**9**)
anthocyanidins (**10**)
proanthocyanidins (**11**)

(+)-gallocatechin (**12**)
(-)-epigallocatechin (**13**)
flavan-3,4-diols (**14**)
type B proanthocyanidins (**15**)
type A proanthocyanidins (**16**)
procyanidins (**17**)
tannins (**18**)
anthocyanins (**19**)
DL-catechin (**20**)
(-)-gallocatechin (**21**)
(-)-epigallocatechin (**22**)
(-)-gallocatechin gallate (**22'**)
(-)-epigallocatechin gallate (**23**)
procyanidin B2 (**24**)
procyanidins B2 (**25**)
3-(3-hydroxyphenyl)propionic acid (**26**)
5-(3,'4,'5'-trihydroxyphenyl)-γ-valerolactone (**27**)
5-(3,'4'-dihydroxyphenyl)-γ-valerolactone (**28**)
rutin (**29**)
3-(3,4-dihydroxyphenyl) propionic acid (**30**)
3-(phenyl)propionic acid (**31**)
3-(4-hydroxy-3-methoxyphenyl)propionic acid (**32**)
pyrogallol (**33**)
pyrocatechol (**34**)
1-(3,'4,'5')-trihydroxyphenyl-3-(2','4','6''-trihydroxy)propan-2-ol (**35**)
1-(3,'4')-dihydroxyphenyl-3-(2','4','6''-trihydroxy)propan-2-ol (**36**)
5-(3,4,5)-trihydroxyphenyl-g-valeric acid (**37**)
5-(3,4)-dihydroxyphenyl-g-valeric acid (**38**)
5-(3,4)-dihydroxyphenyl-g-valeric acid (39)
3-methoxy-4-hydroxyphenylacetic acid (**40**)
3-hydroxyphenylhydracrylic acid (**41**)
4-hydroxybenzoic acid (**42**)
hippuric acid (**43**)
malic acid (**44**)

procyanidin B1 (**45**)
rosmarinic acid (**46**)
procyanidin C1 (**47**)
apigenin (**48**)
ellagic acid (**49**)

AD:	Alzheimer's disease
BB:	brush border
BDNF:	brain-derived neurotrophic factor
BVRT:	Benton visual retention test
bw:	body weight
CBG:	cytosolic β-glucosidase
COMT:	catechol-*O*-methyltransferase
CPE:	cocoa pod extract
CVDs:	cardiovascular diseases
EC_{50}:	50% effective concentration
eNOS:	endothelial nitric oxide synthase
HPC:	hippocampus
IST:	Isaacs set test
LPH:	lactase-phlorizin hydrolase
MCAO:	middle cerebral artery occlusion
MMSE:	mini mental state examination
NOS:	nitric oxide synthase
PD:	Parkinson's disease
PPO:	polyphenol oxydase
ROS:	reactive oxygen species
Rz:	roughness value
SGLT1	sodium-dependent glucose transporter
SULTs:	sulfonotrasnferases
SVZ:	subventricular zone
UGT:	uridine-5'-diphosphate glucuronosyltransferase
UV:	ultraviolet
UVB:	ultraviolet B
WHO:	World Health Organization.

1. Introduction

Cacao is known for its use in chocolate and derived products manufacturing. Cacao seeds are fermented, dry and roasted in order to produce the particular flavor and aroma characteristic of chocolate [1]. Nutritionally, cacao and derived-products are natural sources of biologically active substances with health related effects, such as flavonoids ((-)-epicatechin (**1**), (+)-catechin (**2**), and oligomeric procyanidins (**3**)). The two main flavonoids in cacao, (-)-epicatechin (**1**) and (+)-catechin (**2**), are absorbed in the small intestine, where the aglycone is released and, thereafter the residual flavonoid is sulphated, glucorinated or methylated and, enters to the mesenteric circulation. Oligomeric procyanidins (**3**) are poorly absorbed in the small intestine, but they reach the colon, where they are metabolized by the gut microbiota producing phenolic acids [2, 3]. Studies indicate that cacao-flavonoids (**4**) consumption positively affects the endothelial function, blood pressure, and cholesterol level. In addition, flavonoids (**4**) perform neuroprotective function by reducing oxidation of proteins, and lipid peroxidation, preventing the generation of reactive oxygen species (ROS) and stimulating neuronal regeneration. In this Chapter, the potential function of dietary flavonoids (**4**) to improve cognitive health, neurodegenerative diseases and delay of senescence, is highlighted.

1.1. *Theobroma cacao*

Theobroma cacao is a tropical tree belonging to the Sterculiaceae family, widely distributed in the Western Hemisphere from 18°N Mexico southern to 15°S Amazon forest southern edge [4, 5, 6]. The word cacao is derived from Mayan word *kakaw* and from the chocolate-related Nahuatl term *cacahuatl*. In 1737, Linnaeus named the cocoa tree as *Theobroma cacao* which means “cacao, food of the gods” [7]. The cacao tree was cultivated and consumed by the Mayas in Central America as early as 600 BC [8]; cacao seeds were used to make a beverage flavored with chili, vanilla, honey and annatto described by Aztec Emperor Montezuma as "a divine drink, which builds up resistance and fights fatigue" [9]. This beverage was also associated with wealth and power, moreover, it was used as a gift in funeral ceremonies of dignitaries and as currency [5, 7]. The discovery of America and then its colonization, facilitated the spreading of cacao through Europe, Indonesia, West Indies and West Africa, the last one became a producer out of America. From the 16th century to the19th century, cacao was consumed as a drink only by social elites, and it was not until the late 19th century that it was consumed as solid food and distributed to the general public [8].

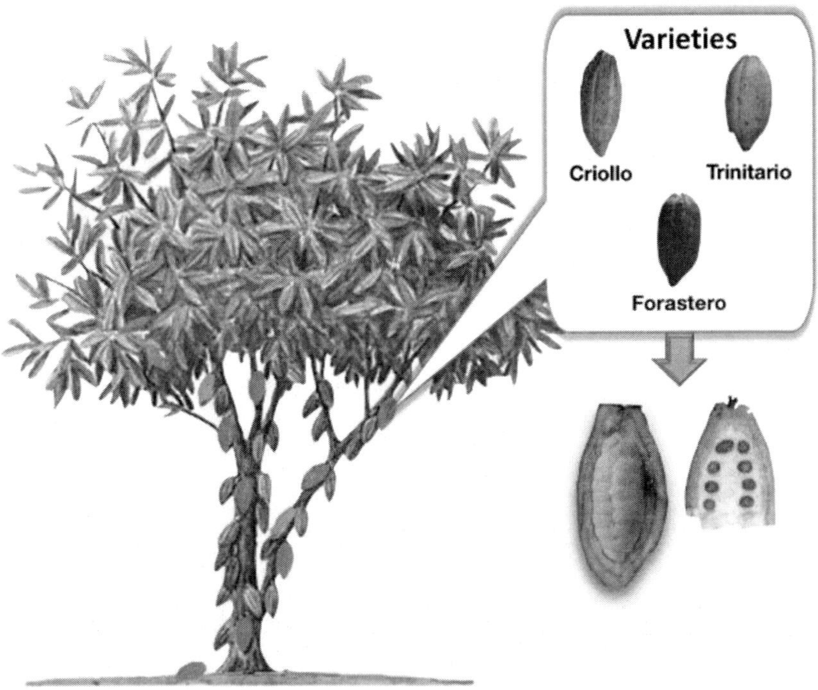

Figure 1. *Theobroma cacao* tree, fruit (varieties), seeds and pod husk.

Cacao bean attributes, such as size, chemical composition, color, flavor and aroma among others vary considerably depending on its genotype, geographical, and agro-climatic conditions during cultivation and the post-harvesting processing [10]. Three main cultivars of cacao are used to make cocoa and chocolate, Criollo *(T. cacao* var *cacao*), Forastero (*T. cacao* var. *sphaerocarpum*) and Trinitario (Figure 1). The Criollo variety is recognized as extra fine cacao due to the slight color of fresh cotyledons and its nutty flavor; it is highly prized and rare, only 5-10% of chocolates are made with this variety [10, 11]. The Forastero variety produced pods of different shapes due to crossings between all varieties; thus, its cotyledons might present tones from purple to dark brown, it also present a strong flavor, slightly bitterness, and higher fat content compared to Criollo, the Forastero variety is used for 80% of world chocolate production. The last variety is Trinitario or Deltano which adopted its name because it was firstly produced in Trinidad y Tobago [5]. It is a hybrid produced from cross-breeding of Criollo with Forastero resulting in cacao beans with a special flavor, used in about 10-15% of chocolate production [11].

2. Flavonoids of Cacao

Phenolic compounds are secondary metabolites of plants that have at least one aromatic ring in which hydroxyl groups are attached; being their principal function the protection against microorganisms, insects, and environmental factors (ultraviolet (UV) radiation, high temperature among others). Cacao polyphenols are stored in the pigment cells of the cotyledons; flavonoids constitute the most important phenolic compounds in cacao [6, 12]. Phenolic compounds are classified as flavonoids and non-flavonoids compounds [13]. Flavonoids (**4**) comprise a group of secondary plant constituents widespread in nature; they consist of 15 carbons with two aromatic rings connected by a three-carbon bridge; they mainly occur as free aglycones, such as galloyl ester or as oligomers. All flavonoids are derived from L-phenylalanine, due to diverse transformations in the phenylpropanoid pathway and forming the flavonoid family comprised by flavones (**5**), flavonols (**6**), flavan-3-ols (**7**), isoflavones (**8**), flavanones (**9**), and anthocyanidins (**10**), which are the main subclasses of flavonoids (Figure 2) [1, 14, 15].

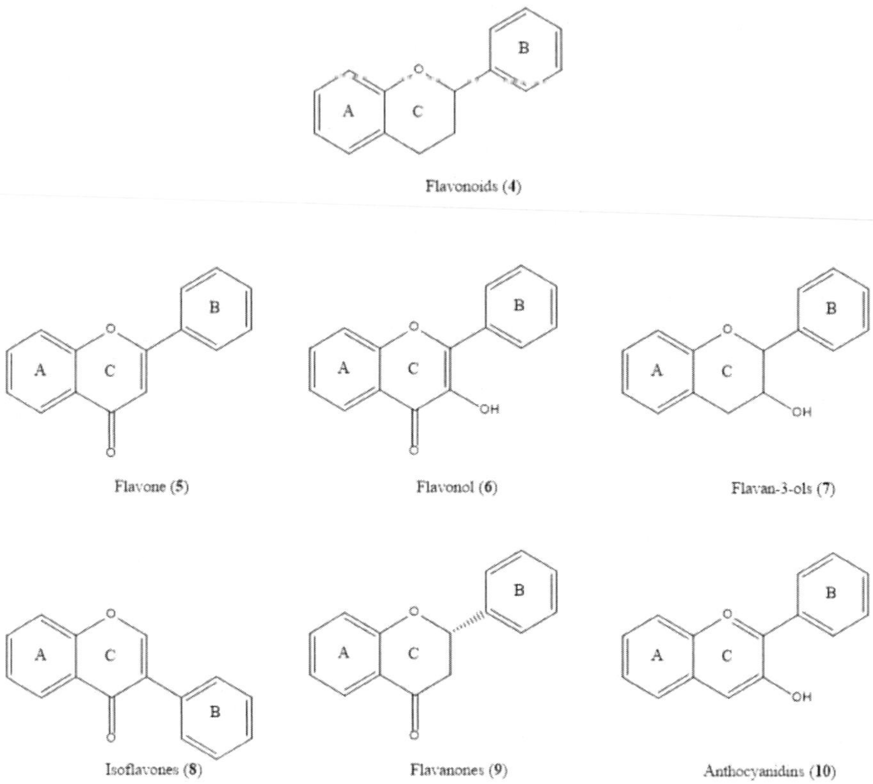

Figure 2. Structures of different types of flavonoids (**4-10**).

Cacao has been reported as a rich source of dietary flavonoids, and its content per serving is higher than the content in teas and red wine [4]. Among cacao polyphenols three main groups of flavonoids can be distinguished: flavan-3-ols (**7**) or catechins (**2'**) (37%), anthocyanins (**19**) (4%) and proanthocyanidins (11) (58%). The main cacao catechin (**2'**) is (-)-epicatechin (**1**) (up to 35%) followed by small amounts of (+)-catechin (**2**), and traces of (+)-gallocatechin (**12**), and (-)-epigallocatechin (**13**) (Figure 3) [6, 16]. Proanthocyanidins (11), also known as condensed tannins are mostly flavan-3,4-diols (**14**), type B proanthocyanidins (**15**) (Figure 3) are formed by (+)-catechin (**2**) and (-)-epicatechin (**1**) monomers by oxidative coupling between the C-4 of the upper monomer and the C-6 and the C-8 of the adjacent lower or extension unit to create oligomers or polymers. On the other hand, type A proanthocyanidins (**16**) (Figure 3) have an additional ether bond between C-2 in the B-ring of one monomer and C-7 in the A-ring of the other monomer. The most abundant type proanthocyanidins (**11**) are those constituted exclusively of (-)-epicatechin (1) as the main subunit extension [1, 6, 14].

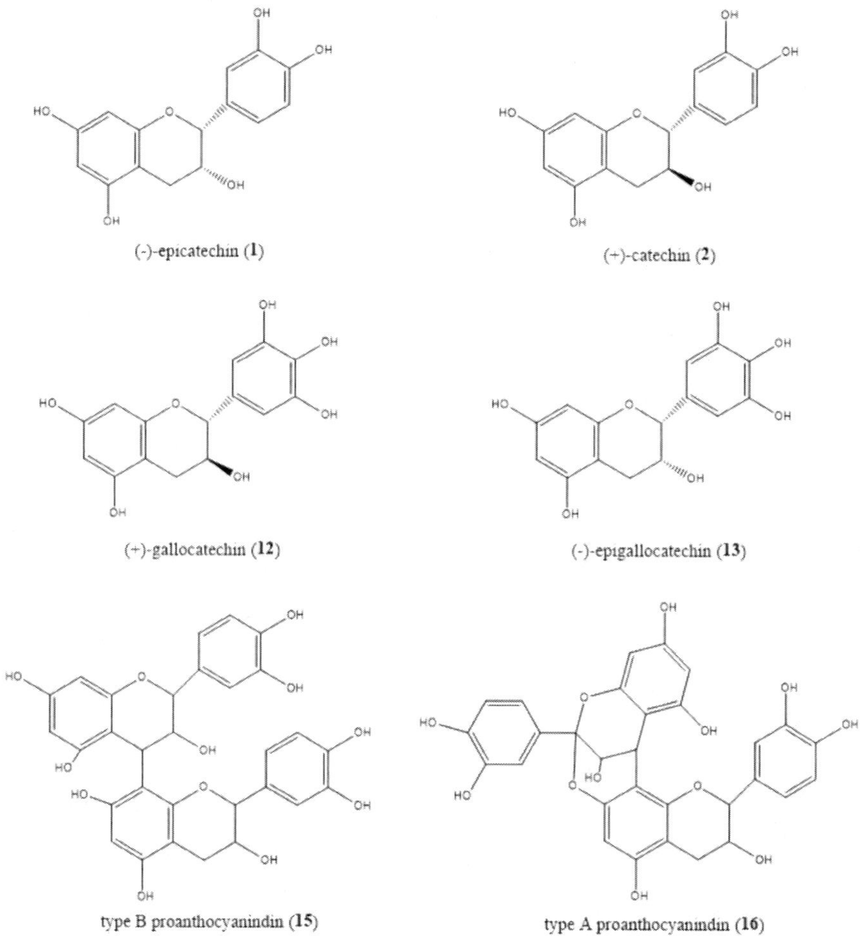

Figure 3. Some of the principal flavonoids (**1, 2, 12, 13, 15**, and **16**) present in cacao.

2.1. Effect of Cacao Bean Processing on Flavonoids

Cacao beans in their natural state have a high concentration of flavonoids making them practically inedible because of the astringency an excessive bitter flavor [18]. During cacao processing to manufacture chocolate and cacao derived-products significant degradations of flavonoids (**4**) occur. Flavonoids (**4**) decrease from 100% to 10%; fermentation, drying and, roasting temperature are the factors involved in the reduction of flavonoids (**4**) content in cacao seeds [4, 18]. Defatted and dry mass of fresh cacao beans have soluble polyphenols in a range of 15-20%, which is equivalent to 6% in air-dried and non-defatted cacao beans [6]. During fermentation cacao polyphenols undergo biochemical oxidation (polyphenol oxidase (PPO); condensing flavonoids, such as (-)-epicatechin (**1**), and (+)-catechin (**2**) into procyanidins (**17**) and insoluble tannins (**18**)) [6]. Epicatechin and soluble polyphenols are reduced to approximately 10 to 20%, proanthocyanidins (**11**) decrease 3- to -5 times and anthocyanins (**19**) disappear during fermentation [12, 16]. In addition, it has been reported that the unfermented fresh cacao and sun-dried beans decrease in 50% its epicatechin (**1'**) content. After fermentation, the cacao beans are dried and roasted until reaching 7% of moisture. Djikeng *et al.* [19] determined, on fermented cacao beans, the effect of traditional roasting (cooking pot at 200-220°C) and oven roasting (180°C); not finding significant differences between methods, moreover, a significant reduction of polyphenolic during roasting was found, this reduction was increased in a direct way by the roasting time.

3. Metabolism of Cacao Flavonoids

Cacao derived-products and chocolate, both rich in flavonoids, are recognized for their medicinal attributes and their biological activity related to health benefits [20]. More than 150 medicinal uses of different parts of cacao (bean, bark, butter, flower, fruit pulp and leaf) are mentioned in the *Badianus Manuscript*, *Florentine Codex* and *Princeton Codex* historical texts [4]. Improving endothelial function and reducing pro-inflammatory mediators are some of the health benefits reported for flavonoid-rich cacao products consumption. Some authors attribute their health benefits to the bioavailability, absorption, distribution, and metabolism of dietary flavonoids (**4**) intake [4, 20]. It has been reported that stereochemistry of flavonoids (*e.g.,* isomerization, monomer bonding type, and degree of polymerization), flavonoid-flavonoid interaction, flavonoid-food matrix interaction and flavonoid-gut microbiota interaction has animpact not only on the absorption rate, but also on the biological action towards the targeted tissues [21].

Molecular size, solubility, chemical structure and the food matrix composition are determinant properties for the absorption and the metabolism of flavonoids (**4**). The chemical structure and the degree of glycosylation, acylation or polymerization that flavonoids (**4**) might present are crucial to their metabolism [11]. The bioavailability of flavonoids (**4**) depends on their absorption, and metabolism at the gastrointestinal tract, their distribution through cells and tissues and the tissue metabolism after absorption. Some studies reported that flavan-3-ols (**7**) and procyanidins (**17**) are stable during gastric transit; allowing their presence at high concentrations in the gastrointestinal tract. High concentrations of low molecular weight flavonols (**6**), monomer, dimers, trimers and tetramers, have been found in blood, having better possibilities to reach the targeted organ in the body [22, 23, 24].

3.1. Digestion and Absorption of Cacao Flavonoids

Bioavailability studies of flavonoids (**4**) and procyanidins (**17**) have demonstrated that in general monomeric units are readily absorbed in the small intestine, whereas polymeric procyanidins (**17**) reach the colon where they are metabolized by the gut microbiota producing phenolic acids [25, 26]. The digestive process of flavonoids begins in the mouth, where flavonoids (**4**) and procyanidins (**17**) groups are bind to salivy, rich in proline proteins, to elicit the characteristic astringent flavor. The flavonoid-proline protein bind degree depends strongly on the chemical structure of the flavonoids (**4**) monomeric units, rather than on the size of the molecule [1, 11, 27]. During the digestion process, a high proportion of flavonoid oligomers (procyanidins (**17**)) are hydrolyzed into dimer and monomer units due to the acidic environment of the gastric environment, dimeric and monomeric flavonoids (**4**) are not affected by the jejune alkaline pH conditions (pH 8.5). Thus, these molecules reached, in an intact way the small intestine with absorption enhancing rates between 22% and 55% [23]. Once flavonoids (**4**) reach the small intestine, those which are glycosylated break the aglycone bond as a result of enzymatic activity. There are two possible routs by which the glucoside conjugates are hydrolyzed and the resultant aglycone is released these two alternatives are "lactase-phlorizin hydrolase (LPH)/diffusion" and "transport/cytosolic beta-glucosidase (CBG)" [3]. The first path way, in which the glycosylated flavonoid is hydrolyzed is through lactase-phlorizin hydrolase (LPH) located in the brush border (BB) of the small intestine epithelial cells. LPH displays substrate specificity for flavonoid-*O*-β-D-glucosides; the released aglycone enters to the epithelial cells by passive diffusion, due to its proximity to the cellular membrane and to its increased lipophilicity [3, 14, 28]. The alternative pathway to hydrolyze the glycosylated flavonoid is through cytosolic *β*-glucosidase (CBG) for polar glycosides within the epithelial cells [29]. For the CBG hydrolysis activity to occur it is necessary that the polar glucosides be transported into the epithelial cells possibly through the involvement of the active sodium-dependent glucose transporter (SGLT1); although this process is currently unclear [3].

After the aglycone is released and prior it reaches the blood stream, it is sulphated, glucoronited and methylated, through the respective action of sulfonotrasnferases (SULTs), uridine-5'-diphosphate glucuronosyltransferase (UGT), and catechol-*O*-methyltransferase (COMT) [3, 14, 26]. Once in the mesenteric circulation, the metabolites of conjugated flavonoids reach the liver, where they can be led to phase II metabolism with further conversions and certain recycling, of these conjugated metabolites, back to the small intestine, through bile excretion [3, 11].

3.2. Flavonoid Metabolization by Gut Microbiota

The studies analyzing the microbial degradation of flavonoids have been assay *in vitro, ex situ* models using a single bacteria species, mixed culture models, human gut microbiota, or pig inoculum (microbiota composition is similar to that of humans in most species) and *in vivo* preclinical studies and clinical trials. Microbiota can hydrolyze different molecules such as glycosides, glucuronides, sulfates, amides, esters, and lactones [25]. According to the studies, most of the dietary flavonoids are absorbed in the small intestine, substantial quantities reach the large intestine [30, 31, 32, 33], where the colonic microbiota breakdown the conjugated moieties, leading to the releasing of the aglycones, which undergo to ring fission to produce smaller molecules, such as phenolic acids and hydroxycinnamates. The proposed pathway of the microbial metabolism of flavonoids is presented in Figure 4.

In regard to flavonoid catabolism of gut microbiota, van't Slot and Humpf [25] using pig cecum model investigated the metabolization of (+)-catechin (**2**), (-)-catechin (**1**), DL-catechin (**20**), (-)-epicatechin (**1**), (-)-gallocatechin (**21**), (-)-epigallocatechin (**13**), (-)-gallocatechin gallate (**22**), (-)-epigallocatechin gallate (**23**), and procyanidin B2 (**24**), for their stereochemistry differences, hydroxylation patterns, and types of bound moieties; founding that monomers are degraded faster than oligomers such as procyanidins B2 (**25**), which resist much longer and are available to exhibit local effects in the gut. In addition they found that microbiota does not distinguish between isomers since there were no differences in concentration-time profiles of the resulting metabolites, such as 3-(3-hydroxyphenyl)propionic acid (**26**), 5-(3,'4,'5'-dihydroxyphenyl)-γ-valerolactone (**27**), and 5-(3,'4'-hydroxyphenyl)-γ-valerolactone (**28**) (Figure 4).

Ekbatan *et al.* [35] characterized the biotransformation of a mixture of pure polyphenols and rutin (**29**), to their microbial metabolites, after 24 hours, simulating the human intestinal microbial ecosystem by using a dynamic gastrointestinal multi-reactor simulator, founding that microbiota metabolized the phenolic compounds into 3-(3,4-dihydroxyphenyl) propionic acid (**30**), 3-(phenyl)propionic acid (**31**), and 3-(4-hydroxy-3-methoxyphenyl)propionic acid (**32**).

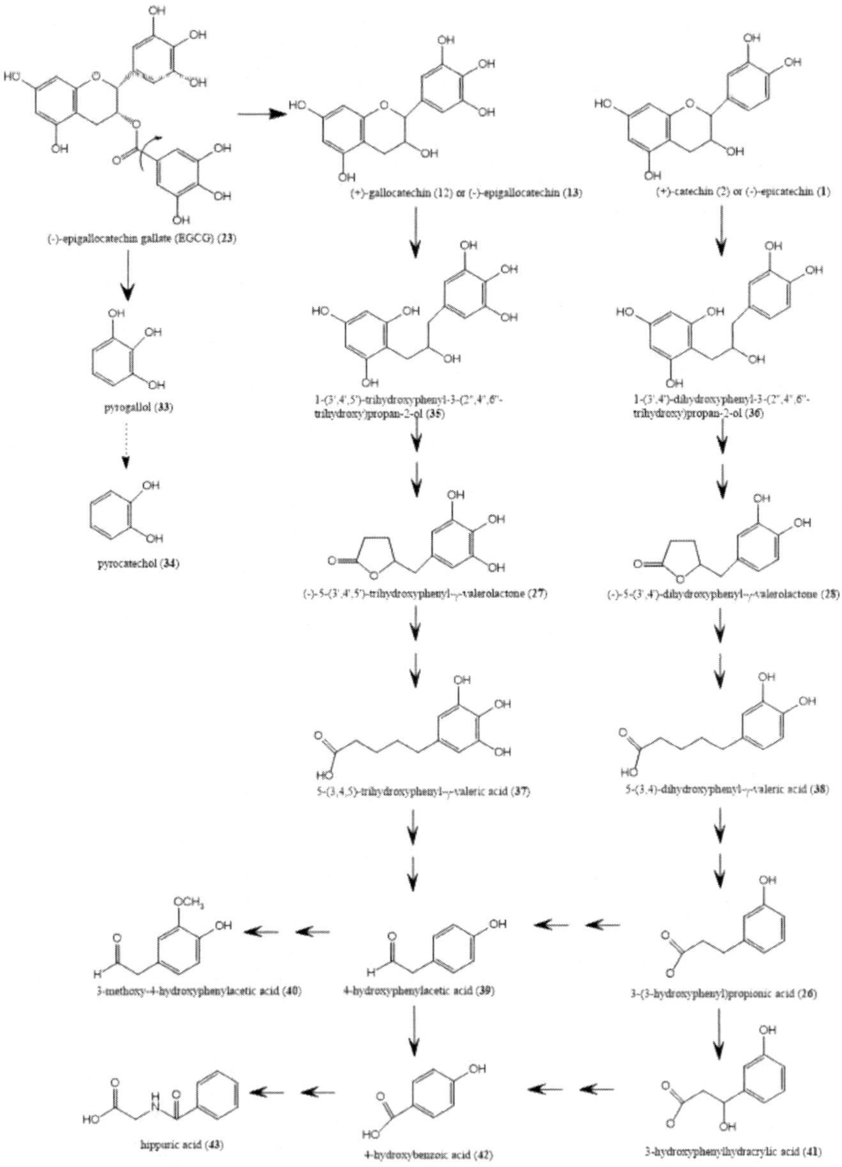

Figure 4. Gut microbiota catabolism of flavonoids (Proposed metabolism, Adapted from Crozier et al. [3] and Chen H, Sang S (2014) [34]).

4. Health Related Effects of Cacao Flavonoids

The epigenetic alterations in chronic pathologies are mainly triggered by oxidative stress and inflammation causing homeostasis imbalance [36]. World Health Organization (WHO) statistics, reported that 35.6 million people worldwide suffer from dementia [37]. Aging is characterized by a progressive systematic dysfunction of nearly all organs and tissues, leading to impaired function and increased vulnerability to environmental challenges that increased death risk. This deterioration not only result in the reduction of physical activity and quality of life, but it is also the primary risk factor for major human pathologies including cardiovascular diseases (CVDs), cancer, diabetes, sarcopenia, and neurodegenerative diseases such as Alzheimer's disease (AD). The common denominators of aging in different organisms are genomic instability, telomere attrition, epigenetic alterations, loss of proteostasis, deregulated nutrient sensing, mitochondrial dysfunction, cellular senescence, stem cell exhaustion, and altered intercellular communication, which have been studied to know their contributions to aging with the final goal to identify pharmaceutical targets to improve human health during aging [38, 39].

Healthy aging has been related to lifestyle, good nutrient balance and a higher intake of food-derived molecules also known as phytochemicals or bioactive compounds. These molecules have the potential to extend life span and to prevent or reduce the risk of chronic diseases [40]. Among these flavonoid molecules can be found and, as it was mentioned before, they possess several biological activities that have certain influence on metabolic and physiological human processes. Cacao is one food which could promote healthy aging; since it has a high content of flavonoids, mainly epicatechin (**1'**) (43.270 mg/kg fruit fresh weight); these effects can be seen in Figure 5. Studies have related epicatechin (**1'**) as the primarily responsible for the beneficial effects of dietary cacao products, including promoting skeletal muscle and vascular function and combating oxidative stress [41, 42, 43, 44]. Thus, the biomedical, biotechnological and pharmaceutical areas have focused on flavonoids as a potential source of natural drugs to treat diseases aging-related processes [45].

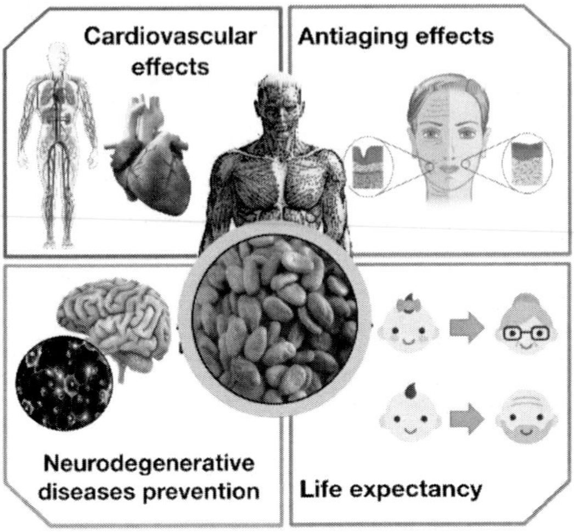

Figure 5. Age-related effect of cacao consumption.

4.1. Cacao and Improvements in Life Expectancy

The age-related effect of cacao has been studied since recent data from epidemiological studies indicated that people living on the San Blas Island of Panama, who consume large amounts of cacao beverages daily, have lower incidence of diabetes, ischemic heart disease, stroke and a remarkably longer lifespan compared to those who live in Panama City. Those beneficial effects disappeared when people migrated from the island to the city reducing the amount of cacao consumption [41, 46, 47]. Kirschbaum [48] reported that chocolate intake (4 kg chocolate/50 kg body weight (bw)) extended by 4 years the average life expectancy in humans. Other study has demonstrated that dietary intake of cocoa or chocolate can improve inflammation, blood pressure, blood vessel function and insulin sensitivity, all of which are related to the aging process [49].

Moreover, preclinical studies have reported that long-term intake of cocoa polyphenolic extract increased the lifespan in aged rats [44, 50, 51]. Si *et al.* [52] researched the beneficial effect of epicatechin (**1'**), finding that 0.25% of this phytochemical, in drinking water, and decreased mortality of diabetic mice after 15 weeks of treatment. In addition, it was found that epicatechin (**1'**) do not altered blood glucose, food intake or body weight gains; suggesting that epicatechin (**1'**) increment of mouse survival is not related to amelioration of hyperglycemia or modulation of calorie intake and metabolism. Similar results on the effect of epicatechin (**1'**) intake were observed in *Drosophila,* administered with 0.01 - 8 mmol/L of epicatechin (**1'**) incorporated into its diet. The same effect of lifespan extension has been observed in *Caenorhabditis elegans* [53].

4.2. Cacao Effects on Improvement of Cognitive Function, and Prevention of Neurodegenerative Disease

Preclinical studies revealed that a 5 months' treatment with a diet rich in polyphenols, dry fruits and cocoa induced neurogenesis in the hippocampus and subventricular zone of adult mice and was able to prevent the neuropathology and cognitive impairment related to the age in wild type (WT) and in a mouse model of Alzheimer's disease (AD). The results support the possibility that polyphenols counteract or slow down cognitive decline during ageing and neurological diseases such as Alzheimer's disease (AD) [54, 55].

Epidemiological studies reported that dietary habits, specially the consumption of antioxidants can influence the incidence of neurodegenerative disorders such as Alzheimer's disease (AD) and Parkinson's disease (PD). Bisson *et al.* [50] evaluated the effect of long-term administration of a cocoa polyphenolic extract on cognitive performances in aged rats; observing an improvement in cognitive performances in light extinction and water maze paradigm. Increased lifespan and preserved high urinary free dopamine levels when rats were administered with cocoa polyphenolic extract at a dose of 24 mg/kg per day during 15 to 27 months were also observed. The results suggest that the beneficial effects exerted by cocoa extract are related to phenolics contained in cacao and their antioxidant activity.

Mastraiacovo *et al.* [56] found that daily consumption of cocoa flavanols (**33**) can improve cognitive function in cognitively intact elderly individuals. The study was carried out in 3 groups which received different doses of cacao flavanols (**7**); high (993 mg), medium (520 mg), and low (48 mg) administered daily in a beverage. After 8 weeks the groups treated with high and medium doses of cacao flavanols (**7**) showed an improvement in performance of neuropsychology tests which measured attentional/executive function and semantic memory. In addition, sensitive markers of cognitive decline and dementia were reduced. Additional to the neurological improvement; cacao consumption also has good effects on some cardiometabolic variables such as blood pressure, insulin resistance, and lipid profile.

Cimini *et al.* [57] reported that cocoa extracts trigger neuroprotection by activating brain-derived neurotrophic factor (BDNF) survival pathway resulting in the concentration of neurite dystrophy attributing this effect to flavonoids (**4**) with antioxidant activity and suggested cocoa consumption might be employed as preventive agent for neurodegeneration. Similar observations were reported by Letenneur *et al.* [58] whose study in the PAQUID (Personnes Agées Quid. elderly quid in English) evaluated the relationship between cognitive function and flavonoid intake, also cognitive malfunction performance was prospectively examined. 1640 subjects were tested four times along 10 years by using the mini mental state examination (MMSE), Benton visual retention test (BVRT) and Isaacs set test (IST). Information about flavonoid (**4**) intake was collected at baseline. The results revealed that subjects with higher flavonoid (**4**) daily intake had a better cognitive performance; suggesting that these food-derived molecules could be associated with better cognitive evolution.

A Norwegian cross-sectional study evaluated the relationship between cognitive function and the intake of chocolate, wine and tea flavonoids (**4**). The subjects (n=2031) aged 70-74 years that consumed three different types of food or beverages with flavonoids (**4**), had a significant improvement in cognitive tests, and had lower prevalence of poor cognitive performance than those who did not consume them. This beneficial relationship was dose-dependent; observing that the maximum effect was when participants consumed ~ 10 g day^{-1} of chocolate and 75-100 mL day^{-1} of wine. No cognitive effect was observed when these foods were consumed independent. Thus, the study suggests that a diet rich in flavonoids (**4**) is associated with a better performance in several cognitive abilities in elderly [59].

Some other studies have focused on the cognitive effects of cacao flavonoids (**4**) to evaluate Alzheimer's disease (AD). The observations suggested that that epicatechin (**1'**) acts directly on the endothelium of the brain vessels by stimulating the activity of the constitutive endothelium nitric oxide synthase (eNOS) to induce vasodilation and thus improve cerebrovascular perfusion [44, 60, 61].

4.3. Cacao and Mediation in Vascular Function

In addition to the cognitive and life expectancy improvement, Flavonoids (**4**)-rich foods exert cardiovascular health benefits. Preclinical studies were carried out administrating 5, 15 or 30 mg kg^{-1} epicatechin (**1'**) on mice as pretreatment 90 min before middle cerebral artery occlusion (MCAO). The effects observed were significantly smaller cerebral lesions and improvement of neurological scores compared to the group without epicatechin. Similar effects were observed when mice were treated with 30 mg kg^{-1} of epicatechin (**1'**) at 3.5 hours after artery occlusion [62].

Buitrago-Lopez *et al.* [63] studied the relationship between the risk reduction of stroke with a high intake of chocolate and observed that the neural lesion caused by the stroke can be reduced when the flavonoids (**4**) intake increases. Some other studies have observed this inversely association between stroke and chocolate flavonoids (**4**) with a reduction of 17% stroke risk in cardiovascular disease (CVD)-free subjects and 47% risk reduction in patients with CVD history [64, 65].

4.4. Cacao and Prevention of Skin Wrinkles

The preventive effect of flavonoids (**4**) on development of skin wrinkles is related to their antioxidant activity. Thus, flavonoids (**4**) have a potential use in cosmetic functional ingredients. In this regard, several studies have examined the relationship of cacao and its antiwrinkle effect. Abdul *et al.* [**66**] studied the antiwrinkle potential of phenolics present in cocoa pod extract (CPE). CPE contains malic acid (**44**), procyanidin B1 (**45**), rosmarinic acid (**46**), procyanidin C1 (**47**), apigenin (**48**), and ellagic acid (**49**). CPE was tested in fibroblast cells in order to determine the effective concentration to maintain the viability of at least 50% of the cells (50% effective concentration (EC_{50})). Twelve panelists were treated with a gel containing CPE. After 3 weeks of gel application, the skin wrinkles were reduced 1.23%, after 5 weeks the wrinkles reduction was 1.59%. No toxic effects were observed after gel application. These results suggest that CPE may be useful for antiwrinkle products development. In addition, CPE exhibit action against elastase and collagenase enzymes, high inhibition towards tyrosine enzyme, induced the proliferation of human fibroblast cells, and potential ultraviolet B (UVB) sunscreen protection [67].

Yoon *et al.* [68] evaluated the effect of oral supplementation with cocoa flavonoids (**4**) on cutaneous photo-aged Korean women with visible facial wrinkles. The participants were randomly assigned to receive a placebo beverage or a cocoa beverage (320 mg of total cocoa flavanols (**7**) per day). Wrinkles, skin elasticity, and hydration skin were measured at baseline, 12 and 24 weeks. The observable effects of cacao consumption were, change in the average roughness value (Rz) at week 24, and reduction of the gross elasticity. Skin hydration and barrier integrity between groups did not change. This study suggests that cocoa flavonoids (**4**) had a positive effect on facial wrinkles of elasticity preventing the progression of photo-aging.

CONCLUSION

The use of flavonoids (**4**) from cacao to prevent chronic diseases or to improve some of their complications mainly related to the oxidative stress and aging, had been research in several studies highlighting that an improvement of diet, and an incorporation of flavonoids (**4**) into the long term with a continuous intake can improve aging related problems. Cacao flavonoids (**4**) consumption can induce neurogenesis in the hippocampus (HPC) and subventricular zone (SVZ), prevent the neuropathology and cognitive impairment related to the age, improving stroke lesions. These health benefits make cacao a suitable alternative to treat aging-related problems.

REFERENCES

[1] Ellam S, Williamson G. Cocoa and human health. *Annu Rev Nutr* 33, 105-128, 2013.

[2] Cardona F, Andrés-Lacueva C, Tulipani S, Tinahones FJ. Queipo-Ortuño MI. Benefits of polyphenols on gut microbiota and implications in human health. *Journal of Nutritional Biochemistry* 24(8), 1415-1422, 2013.

[3] Crozier A, Del Rio D, Clifford MN. Bioavailability of dietary flavonoids and phenolic compounds. *Mol Aspects Med* 31(6), 446-467, 2010.

[4] Hii CL, Law CL, CL, Suzannah S, Misnawi, Cloke M. Polyphenols in cocoa (*Theobroma cacao* L.). *Asian Journal of Food and Agro-Industry* 2(4), 702-722, 2009.

[5] Rangel-Fajardo MA, Zavaleta-Mancera HA, Córdova-Téllez L, López-Andrade AP, Delgado-Alvarado A, Vidales-Fernández I, Villegas-Monter Á. Anatomía e histoquímica de la semilla del cacao (*Theobroma cacao* L.) criollo mexicano [Anatomy and histochemical of the mexican creole cacao seed (*Theobroma cacao* L.)]. *Rev Fitotec Mex (Fitotecnia Mexicana Journal)* 35(3), 189-197, 2012.

[6] Wollgast J, Anklam W. Review on polyphenols in *Theobroma cacao*: changes in composition during the manufacture of chocolate and methodology for identification and quantification. *Food Research International* 33(6), 423-447, 2000.

[7] Ruzaidi A, Maleyki A, Amin I, Nawalyah, Muhajir AG, Pauliena MBSJ, Muskinah MS. Hypoglycaemic properties of Malaysian cocoa

(*Theobroma cacao*) polyphenols-rich extract. *International Food Research Journal* 15(3), 305-312, 2008.

[8] Vega CC. Kwik-Uribe C. *Theobroma cacao* - An introduction to the plant, its composition, uses, and health benefits. pp. 36-62 (Chapter 2). In: Garti N, Widlak NR (eds). *Butter and Related Compounds*. 2012. Academic Press, USA.

[9] Kim J, K. W. Lee KW, Lee HJ. Cocoa (*Theobroma cacao*) seeds and phytochemicals in human health. pp. 351-360 (Chapter 42). In: Preedy V, Watson R, V. B. Patel V (eds). *Nuts and Seeds in Health and Disease Prevention*. 2011. San Diego, Academic Press, USA.

[10] Pérez GL, Maciel BMM, López JH, Covarrubias FM, López JL, Aguilar G, Pérez JLR, Medina LL, Vargas F. Prevalencia de las enfermedades alérgicas en la Ciudad de México [Prevalence of allergic diseases in the City of Mexico]. *Rev Alerg Mex* 56(3), 72-79, 2009.

[11] Rusconi M, Conti A. *Theobroma cacao* L., the Food of the Gods: a scientific approach beyond myths and claims. *Pharmacol Res* 61(1), 5-13, 2010.

[12] Andújar I, M. Recio MC, Giner RM, Ríos JL. Cocoa polyphenols and their potential benefits for human health. *Oxidative Medicine and Cellular Longevity* 2012, 2012.

[13] Gutiérrez Maydata BA. Chocolate, polifenoles y protección a la salud (Chocolate, polyphenols and health protection). *Acta Farmacéutica Bonaerense* 21(2), 149-152, 2002.

[14] Rio DA. Rodriguez-Mateos A, Spencer JPE, Tognolini M, Borges G, Crozier A. Dietary (poly)phenolics in human health: Structures, bioavailability, and evidence of protective effects against chronic diseases. *Antioxid Redox Signal* 18(14), 1818-1892, 2013.

[15] Scapagnini G, Davinelli S, Di Renzo L, De Lorenzo A, Olarte HH, Micali G, Cicero AF, Gonzalez S. Cocoa bioactive compounds: significance and potential for the maintenance of skin health. *Nutrients* 6(8), 3202-3213, 2014.

[16] Perea-Villamil JA, Cadena-Cala T, Herrera-Ardila J. El cacao y sus productos como fuente de antioxidantes: Efecto del procesamiento

[The cocoa and its products as antioxidant source: Processing effect]. *Revista de la Universidad Industrial de Santander. Salud* 41(2), 128-134, 2009.

[17] Bonvehi JS, Coll. FV. Evaluation of bitterness and astringency of polyphenolic compounds in cocoa powder. *Food Chemistry* 60(3), 365-370, 1997.

[18] Hernández-Hernández C, Viera-Alcaide I, Morales-Sillero AM, J. Fernández-Bolaños J, Rodríguez-Gutiérrez G. Bioactive compounds in Mexican genotypes of cocoa cotyledon and husk. *Food Chemistry* 240, 831-839, 2018.

[19] Djikeng FT, Teyomnou WT, Tenyang N, Tiencheu B, Morfor AT, Touko BAH, Houketchang SN, Boungo GT, Karuna MSL, Ngoufack FZ, Womeni HM. Effect of traditional and oven roasting on the physicochemical properties of fermented cocoa beans. *Heliyon* 4(2), e00533, 2018.

[20] Schinella G, Mosca S, Cienfuegos-Jovellanos E, Pasamar MÁ, Muguerza B, Ramón D, Ríos JL. Antioxidant properties of polyphenol-rich cocoa products industrially processed. *Food Research International* 43(6), 1614-1623, 2010.

[21] Fraga CG, Oteiza P. Dietary flavonoids: Role of (-)-epicatechin and related procyanidins in cell signaling. *Free Radic Biol Med* 51(4), 813-823, 2011.

[22] Rios LY, Bennett RN, Lazarus SA, Rémésy C, Scalbert A, Williamson G. Cocoa procyanidins are stable during gastric transit in humans. *Am J Clin Nutr* 76(5), 1106-1110, 2002.

[23] Spencer JP, Chaudry F, Pannala AS, Srai SK, Debnam E, Rice-Evans C. Decomposition of cocoa procyanidins in the gastric milieu. *Biochem Biophys Res Commun* 272(1), 236-2341, 2000.

[24] Spencer JP, Schroeter H, Shenoy B, Srai SK, Debnam ES, Rice-Evans C. Epicatechin is the primary bioavailable form of the procyanidin dimers B2 and B5 after transfer across the small intestine. *Biochem Biophys Res Commun* 285(3), 588-593, 2001.

[25] Van't Slot G, Humpf HU. Degradation and metabolism of catechin, epigallocatechin-3-gallate (EGCG), and related compounds by the

intestinal microbiota in the pig cecum model. *J Agric Food Chem* 57(17), 8041-8048, 2009.

[26] Vitaglione P, Barone Lumaga R, Ferracane R, Sellitto S, Morelló JR, Reguant Miranda J, Shimoni E, Fogliano V. Human bioavailability of flavanols and phenolic acids from cocoa-nut creams enriched with free or microencapsulated cocoa polyphenols. *Br J Nutr* 109(10), 1832-1843, 2013.

[27] Gallo M, Vinci G, Graziani G, Simone CD, Ferranti P. The interaction of cocoa polyphenols with milk proteins studied by proteomic techniques. *Food Research International* 54(1), 406-415, 2013.

[28] Selma MV, Espín JC, Tomás-Barberán FA. Interaction between phenolics and gut microbiota: role in human health. *J Agric Food Chem* 57(15), 6485-6501, 2009.

[29] Marín L, Miguélez EM, Villar CJ, Lombó F. Bioavailability of dietary polyphenols and gut microbiota metabolism: antimicrobial properties. *Biomed Res Int* 2015;2015:905215. doi: 10.1155/2015/905215.

[30] Kahle K, Kraus M, Scheppach W, Ackermann M, Ridder F, Richling E. Studies on apple and blueberry fruit constituents: do the polyphenols reach the colon after ingestion? *Mol Nutr Food Res* 50(4-5), 418-423, 2006.

[31] Kahle K, Kraus M, Scheppach W, Richling E. Colonic availability of apple polyphenols--a study in ileostomy subjects. *Mol Nutr Food Res* 49(12), 1143-1150, 2005.

[32] Jaganath IB, Mullen W, Edwards CA, Crozier A. The relative contribution of the small and large intestine to the absorption and metabolism of rutin in man. *Free Radic Res* 40(10), 1035-1046, 2006.

[33] Marks SC, Mullen W, Borges G, Crozier A. Absorption, metabolism, and excretion of cider dihydrochalcones in healthy humans and subjects with an ileostomy. *J Agric Food Chem* 57(5), 2009-2015, 2009.

[34] Chen H, Sang S. Biotransformation of tea polyphenols by gut microbiota. *Journal of Functional Foods* 7, 26-42, 2014.

[35] Ekbatan SS, Sleno L, Sabally K, Khairallah J, Azadi B, Rodes L, Prakash S, Donnelly DJ, Kubow S. Biotransformation of polyphenols in a dynamic multistage gastrointestinal model. *Food Chemistry* 204, 453-462, 2016.

[36] Corbi G, Conti V, Davinelli S, Scapagnini G, Filippelli A, Ferrara N. Dietary phytochemicals in neuroimmunoaging: A new therapeutic possibility for humans? *Front Pharmacol* 13;7:364. eCollection 2016.

[37] Latif R. Flavonoids as novel neuroprotective nutraceuticals. *Saudi Journal for Health Sciences* 4(1), 1-4, 2015.

[38] López-Otín C, Blasco MA, Partridge L, Serrano M, Kroemer G. The hallmarks of aging. *Cell* 153(6), 1194-1217, 2014.

[39] Murphy SL, Xu J, Kochanek KD, Curtin SC, Arias E. Deaths: Final Data for 2015. *Natl Vital Stat Rep* 66(6), 1-75, 2017.

[40] Si H, Liu D. Dietary antiaging phytochemicals and mechanisms associated with prolonged survival. *J Nutr Biochem* 25(6), 581-591, 2014.

[41] Hollenberg NK, Fisher ND. Is it the dark in dark chocolate? *Circulation* 116(21), 2360-2362, 2007.

[42] Moreno-Ulloa A, Nogueira L, Rodriguez A, Barboza J, Hogan MC, Ceballos G, Villarreal F, Ramirez-Sanchez I. Recovery of indicators of mitochondrial biogenesis, oxidative stress, and aging with (-)-epicatechin in senile mice. *J Gerontol A Biol Sci Med Sci* 70(11), 1370-1378, 2015.

[43] Nogueira L, Ramirez-Sanchez I, Perkins GA, Murphy A, Taub PR, Ceballos G, Villarreal FJ, Hogan MC, Malek MH. (-)-Epicatechin enhances fatigue resistance and oxidative capacity in mouse muscle. *J Physiol* 589(Pt 18), 4615-4631, 2011.

[44] Schroeter H, Heiss C, Balzer J, Kleinbongard P, Keen CL, Hollenberg NK, Sies H, Kwik-Uribe C, Schmitz HH, Kelm M. (-)-Epicatechin mediates beneficial effects of flavanol-rich cocoa on

vascular function in humans. *Proc Natl Acad Sci USA* 103(4), 1024-1029, 2006.

[45] Bernatova I. Biological activities of (-)-epicatechin and (-)-epicatechin-containing foods: Focus on cardiovascular and neuropsychological health. *Biotechnol Adv* 36(3), 666-681, 2018.

[46] Bayard V, Chamorro F, Motta J, Hollenberg NK. Does flavanol intake influence mortality from nitric oxide-dependent processes? Ischemic heart disease, stroke, diabetes mellitus, and cancer in Panama. *International journal of Medical Sciences* 4(1), 53-58, 2007.

[47] Hollenberg NK, Martinez G, McCullough M, Meinking T, Passan D, Preston M, Rivera A, Taplin D, Vicaria-Clement M. Aging, acculturation, salt intake, and hypertension in the Kuna of Panama. *Hypertension* 29(1 Pt 2), 171-176, 1997.

[48] Kirschbaum J. Effect on human longevity of added dietary chocolate. *Nutrition* 14(11-12), 869, 1998.

[49] Ding EL, Hutfless SM, Ding X, Girotra S. Chocolate and prevention of cardiovascular disease: a systematic review. *Nutr Metab (Lond)* 2006 Jan 3;3:2, 2006.

[50] Bisson JF, Nejdi A, Rozan P, Hidalgo S, Lalonde R, Messaoudi M. Effects of long-term administration of a cocoa polyphenolic extract (Acticoa powder) on cognitive performances in aged rats. *Br J Nutr* 100(1), 94-101, 2008.

[51] Holt RR, Actis-Goretta L, Momma TY, Keen CL. Dietary flavanols and platelet reactivity. *J Cardiovasc Pharmacol* 47(Suppl 2), S187-S196; discussion S206-S209, 2006.

[52] Si H, Fu Z, Babu PV, Zhen W, Leroith T, Meaney MP, Voelker KA, Jia Z, Grange RW, Liu D. Dietary epicatechin promotes survival of obese diabetic mice and Drosophila melanogaster. *J Nutr* 141(6), 1095-1100, 2011.

[53] Sunagawa T, Shimizu T, Kanda T, Tagashira M, Sami M, Shirasawa T. Procyanidins from apples (*Malus pumila* Mill.) extend the lifespan of *Caenorhabditis elegans*. *Planta Med* 77(2), 122-1227, 2011.

[54] Fernández-Fernández L, Comes G, Bolea I, Valente T, Ruiz J, Murtra P, Ramirez B, Anglés N, Reguant J, Morelló JR, Boada M,

Hidalgo J, Escorihuela RM, Unzeta M. LMN diet, rich in polyphenols and polyunsaturated fatty acids, improves mouse cognitive decline associated with aging and Alzheimer's disease. *Behav Brain Res* 228(2), 261-271, 2012.

[55] Valente T, Hidalgo J, Bolea I, Ramirez B, Anglés N, Reguant J, Morelló JR, Gutiérrez C, Boada M, Unzeta M. A diet enriched in polyphenols and polyunsaturated fatty acids, LMN diet, induces neurogenesis in the subventricular zone and hippocampus of adult mouse brain. *J Alzheimers Dis* 18(4), 849-65, 2009.

[56] Mastroiacovo D, Kwik-Uribe C, Grassi D, Necozione S, Raffaele A, Pistacchio L, Righetti R, Bocale R, Lechiara MC, Marini C, Claudio Ferri C, Desideri G. Cocoa flavanol consumption improves cognitive function, blood pressure control, and metabolic profile in elderly subjects: the Cocoa, Cognition, and Aging (CoCoA) Study-a randomized controlled trial. *Am J Clin Nutr* 101(3), 538–548, 2015.

[57] Cimini A, Gentile R, D'Angelo B, Benedetti E, Cristiano L, Avantaggiati ML, Giordano A, Ferri C, Desideri G. Cocoa powder triggers neuroprotective and preventive effects in a human Alzheimer's disease model by modulating BDNF signaling pathway. *J Cell Biochem* 114(10), 2209-2220, 2013.

[58] Letenneur L, Proust-Lima C, Le Gouge A, Dartigues JF, Barberger-Gateau P. Flavonoid intake and cognitive decline over a 10-year period. *Am J Epidemiol* 165(12), 1364-1371, 2007.

[59] Nurk E, Refsum H, Drevon CA, Tell GS, Nygaard HA, Engedal K, Smith AD. Intake of flavonoid-rich wine, tea, and chocolate by elderly men and women is associated with better cognitive test performance. *J Nutr* 139(1), 120-127, 2009.

[60] Fisher ND, Sorond FA, Hollenberg NK. Cocoa flavanols and brain perfusion. *J Cardiovasc Pharmacol* 47(Suppl 2), S210-S204, 2006.

[61] Patel AK, Rogers JT, Huang X. Flavanols, mild cognitive impairment, and Alzheimer's dementia. *International Journal of Clinical and Experimental Medicine* 1(2), 181-191, 2008.

[62] Shah ZA, Li RC, Ahmad AS, Kensler TW, Yamamoto M, Biswal S, Doré S. The flavanol (-)-epicatechin prevents stroke damage through

the Nrf2/HO1 pathway. *J Cereb Blood Flow Metab* 30(12), 1951-1961, 2010.

[63] Buitrago-Lopez A, Sanderson J, Johnson L, Warnakula S, Wood A, Di Angelantonio E, Franco OH. Chocolate consumption and cardiometabolic disorders: systematic review and meta-analysis. *BMJ* 2011 Aug 26;343:d4488. doi: 10.1136/bmj.d4488.

[64] Buijsse B, Weikert C, Drogan D, Bergmann M, Boeing H. Chocolate consumption in relation to blood pressure and risk of cardiovascular disease in German adults. *Eur Heart J* 31(13), 1616-1623, 2010.

[65] Rautiainen S, Larsson S, Virtamo J, Wolk A. Total antioxidant capacity of diet and risk of stroke: a population-based prospective cohort of women. *Stroke* 43(2), 335-340, 2012.

[66] Abdul Karim A, Azlan A, Ismail A, Hashim P, Abd Gani SS, Zainudin BH, Abdullah NA. Efficacy of cocoa pod extract as antiwrinkle gel on human skin surface. *J Cosmet Dermatol* 15(3), 283-295, 2016.

[67] Karim AA, Azlan A, Ismail A, Hashim, P, Gani SSA, ainudin BH, N. A. Abdullah NA. Phenolic composition, antioxidant, anti-wrinkles and tyrosinase inhibitory activities of cocoa pod extract. *BMC Complementary and Alternative Medicine* 14(1), 381, 2014.

[68] Yoon HS, Kim JR, Park GY, Kim JE, Lee DH, Lee KW, Chung JH. Cocoa flavanol supplementation influences skin conditions of photo-aged women: A 24-week double-blind, randomized, controlled trial. *J Nutr* 146(1), 46-50, 2016.

In: Natural Anti-Aging Plants …
Editor: Noboru Motohashi
ISBN: 978-1-53616-282-0

Chapter 4

AGING AND HORMONES (ANTIAGING HORMONES)

Noboru Motohashi[1,*] and J. Seetharamappa[2,†]
[1]Meiji Pharmaceutical University, Kiyose-shi, Tokyo, Japan
[2]Department of Chemistry, Karnatak University, Dharwad, India

ABSTRACT

In general, diseases associated with aging are inevitable diseases for humans which are involved in the entire body such as cardiovascular system (heart disease), respiratory system (pneumonia), digestive system (reflux esophagitis), kidney and urinary system (incontinence), nervous system (Alzheimer's disease, Parkinson's disease), bone and motor system (osteoporosis), sensory organ system (senile cataract), degradation of masticatory forces and so on.

Humans will need some treatment for these diseases with age. The reason for this is that elderly people are more likely to suffer from physiological dysfunction with age than young people. Humans must minimize this physiological dysfunction in order to stay fit for the rest of their lives.

* Corresponding Author's E-mail: noborumotohashi@jcom.home.ne.jp.
† Corresponding Author's E-mail: jseetharam97@gmail.com.

As humans age, their hormonal performance may decline, and sometimes even increase, as compared to their younger age. Therefore, humans need to re-set their normal hormone balance, that is, homeostasis (hormone homeostasis), with normal hormone balance, that is, the symptoms associated with insufficient secretion or increased secretion of hormones, or imbalance or increase in hormone balance involved in most important physiological functions. Proper hormonal treatment is thought to regulate, stop or delay changes in hormone production with age.

Therefore, in this Chapter, we mainly described to the representative human growth hormone (HGH), melatonin, thyrotropin, thyroid hormone, calcitonin (CT), dehydroepiandrosterone (DHEA), aldosterone, and estrogen that are currently expected for hormone therapy, and described based on their effects on the physiological functions and the results of epidemiological surveys of each hormone.

Keywords: Human growth hormone (HGH), aging, age-related changes, sex hormones, serum dehydroepiandrosterone sulfate (DS. DHEAS), loop diuretic, bone mineral density (BMD)

Chemical Constituents in Hormones

melantonin (**1**)
thyrotropin (TSH. **2**)
thyroxine (T4. **3**)
triiodothyronine (TIT. T3. **4**)
calcitonin (CT. **5**)
dehydroepiandrosterone sulfate (DS. **6**)
dehydroepiandrosterone (DHEA. **7**)
androgen (**8**)
testosterone (**8.1**)
dihydrotestosterone (DHT. **8.2**)
female hormone (E. estrogen. **9**)
estradiol (E_2. **9.1**)
estriol (**9.2**)
estrone (E_1. **9.3**)
progesterone (**9.4**)

aldosterone (**10**)
furosemide (**11**)
osteocalcin (OC. **12**)
free deoxypyridinoline (**13**)

ABBREVIATIONS

ALP	alkaline phosphatase
Ang II	angiotensin II
ANOVA	analyses of variance
APCCs	aldosterone-producing cell clusters
ARR	aldosterone/renin ratio
BA	bioavailability
BAP	bone-specific alkaline phosphatase
BMD	bone mineral density
BMI	body mass index
r	correlation coefficient
CT	calcitonin
CYP11B2	cytochrome P450 aldosterone synthase
DHEA	dehydroepiandrosterone
DS (DHEAS)	dehydroepiandrosterone sulfate
E	serum estrogen
F	F statistic
FSH	follicle-stimulating hormone
GH	growth hormone
GHRH	growth hormone releasing hormone
GRF	growth hormone releasing factor)
HAS	human serum albumin
HDL cholesterol	high-density lipoprotein cholesterol
HGH	human growth hormone
IGF-1	insulin-like growth factor-1
LDL cholesterol	low-density lipoprotein cholesterol
LH	luteinizing hormone

meq	milli equivalents
NTx	cross-linked *N*-telopeptide of type I collagen
p	significance probability
PA	primary aldosteronism (primary hyperaldosteronism)
PICP	carboxy-terminal propeptide of type I procollagen
PRA	panel-reactive antibody
PTH	parathormone
PTH	parathyroid hormone
RIA	radioimmunoassay
ROS	reactive oxygen species
SASSI	sodiummodulated aldosterone suppression-to-stimulation index
SE	standard error
SH	sex steroid hormone
SHBG	serum sex hormone-binding globulin
TBG	sthyroxine-binding globulin
y	linear transformation
ZG	zona glomerulosa

1. Introduction

The cause and treatment of human aging (pathological aging) is a very long-standing subject. Humans have always had the desire to be healthy and to live longer. It probably goes back to the dawn of humanity a million years ago. The first emperor who achieved Chinese unification around the 3rd century BC sought for immortality. In fact, it is recorded in China's historical book "History" that the first emperor ordered Xoofu to go to the kingdom of Qin to bring in some *immortals* or to bring in *panacea*. In the West, there is an *alchemy spirit drug* called Elixir, an immortal drug as elixir of life [1].

2. ANTIAGING HORMONES

All the humans develop hormone decline (hormone loss) in proportion to their age. The purpose of antiaging therapy is to delay hormonal changes associated with aging, or to suppress aging and restore young body because hormonal changes are involved in aging.

2.1. Human Growth Hormone (HGH) and Insulin-Like Growth Factor-1 (IGF-1)

Human growth hormone (HGH) injection is used in hormone replacement therapy (anti-aging therapy) for the purpose of rejuvenation and anti-aging. According to the experimental results of aged rat, decreased tissue function is associated with decreased rate of protein synthesis. Such changes in tissue function may be caused, in part, by decreased secretion of growth hormone (GH) and insulin-like growth factor 1 (IGF-1).

It is also known that growth hormone releasing hormone (growth hormone releasing factor. GHRH. GRF. somatocrinin), and somatostatin (a peptide hormone that suppresses the secretion of secondary hormones such as growth hormone (GH)) plays an important role in the regulation of growth hormone (GH) secretion. And it has also been found that increased somatostatin release is one of the main causes of decreased growth hormone (GH) secretion with aging.

Based on the above findings, in 1993, a grouop of Department of Physiology and Pharmacology, Bowman Gray School of Medicine, Wake Forest University, NC, USA examined the regulation and role of growth hormone (GH) and insulin-like growth factor 1 (IGF-1) during aging, using a single calorie restriction model. When the somatostatin mRNA level was examined, the old rat decreased the somatostatin mRNA level. However, the amount of somatostatin mRNA bound to polysomes was increased in these aged rats. This means that the translational regulatory mechanism is impaired in old rats. Moderate dietary restriction has been shown to prolong lifespan, has enhanced the amplitude of growth hormone (GH) pulses and the ability of tissues to synthesize proteins. From this aged rat experiment, it is evident that neuroendocrine regulation of growth hormone (GH) secretion plays an important role in the process of aging organisms. Some beneficial effects of moderate dietary restriction were mediated by altering the growth hormone (GH) and insulin-like growth factor 1 (IGF-1) axes [2].

Mean plasma growth hormone (GH) levels differ significantly due to pathophysiological changes and symptoms such as obesity, fasting, exercise, type 1 diabetes, adolescence, *etc*. [3-8].

Although growth hormone (GH) secretion in adults is pulsatile, healthy older adults have decreased total pulsatilse growth hormone (GH) release [3, 4, 9-18].

However, according to some reports, no significant decrease in growth hormone (GH) release with age has been reported, but in other studies the decrease in growth hormone (GH) release is very high and noticeable in women when compared to that(decrease) in men.

A convincing cause for the differences among the above reports with regard to the reduction of growth hormone (GH) release is probably due to other confounding variables such as body weight, nutritional status, sex steroid hormone concentration that may exhibit independent or combined effects for total growth hormone (GH) release and pulsatile growth hormone (GH) release. It is difficult to fully assess the reduction in growth hormone (GH) release as long as the relative role of such factors is not controlled by the effects of at least one or more variables [19, 20].

With respect to circulating growth hormone (GH) molecules, the beating pattern of serum growth hormone (GH) concentration is believed to be due to a spike-like pattern of intermittent growth hormone (GH) secretion combined with specific metabolic clearance (whole body clearance. Sum of liver clearance and liver specific clearance) of both patients and their symptoms.

Thus, changes *either* in the half-life of the secreted growth hormone (GH) molecule or in the frequency, amplitude, mass, and/or duration of the idiopathic growth hormone (GH) secretory burst account for the reported variations in average serum growth hormone (GH) concentrations. From deconvolution analysis (convolution integral) is used to determine these dynamic features from the measurement of mean serum growth hormone (GH) concentrations [19, 20].

Based on the above facts, in 1991, a group of Department of Internal Medicine, Salem Veterans Administration Hospital, Virginia, USA examined the relationship between age and relative obesity with specific negative determinants of frequency and amplitude of growth hormone (GH) secretory burst and the half-life of endogenous growth hormone (GH) in healthy men. Therefore, in this study, in order to control several known confounding variables. A normal adult male group both in the fed state and in the absence of chronic disease, morbid obesity, or sex steroid hormone deficiency was used. The following specific hypotheses could be tested in this healthy male cohort: First, the age acts as an individual specific feature of growth hormone (GH) secretion (secretory burst mass, frequency, amplitude, or duration), or an important determinant of endogenous growth hormone (GH) half-life; Second, the degree of relative obesity, as defined by body mass index (kg/m^2), showed a independently significant relationship between specific growth hormone (GH) secretion and /or clearance parameters; Third, age, and body mass index (BMI) jointly determine growth hormone (GH) secretion rate and /or clearance rate in the clinically healthy non-obese male population.

Deconvolution analysis revealed that the growth hormone (GH) secretory burst frequency decreased significantly with increase in age. On the other hand, growth hormone (GH) secretory burst wave amplitude changed negatively with body mass index (BMI). The calculated half-life of endogenous growth hormone (GH) was adversely affected by age alone, body mass index (BMI) alone, and these two co-effects. These observations were specific because the amount and duration of the growth hormone (GH) secretion burst did not correlate with age, body mass index (BMI), or a combined variable.

The use of more sensitive assay methods, more rigorous deconvoluted integration techniques, and/or more frequent blood sampling to measure serum growth hormone (GH) concentrations can affect the absolute number of bursts detectable growth hormone (GH) secretion. Nevertheless, technical considerations seem unlikely to explain the strong adverse effects of age on growth hormone (GH) secretory burst frequency. This is because growth hormone (GH) secretion burst frequency did not significantly reduce the amplitude or amount of growth hormone (GH) secretion burst only by increasing the age.

Furthermore, in addition to age, body mass index (BMI) and the relative obesity scale were negatively correlated with the daily growth hormone (GH) secretion rate of healthy men. The statistical significance (significance probability (p) = 0.027) of body mass index (BMI) alone was lower when compared to that of the relative obesity scale alone (p = 0.0031). Two variables of body mass index (BMI) and relative obesity scale were jointly very strong negative predictors of daily growth hormone (GH) secretion in healthy men (p = 0.00056; correlation coefficient (r) = -0.78). In fact, over 60% of the daily growth hormone (GH) secretion rate fluctuation was due to the combined effect of age and body mass index (BMI). The daily growth hormone (GH) secretion rate was estimated to decrease by 6-14% per decade with each unit increase in body mass index (BMI). The 24-hour growth hormone (GH) production rate was reduced by 50% each when compared to that (24-hour growth hormone (GH) production rate) of 21-year-old men and 45-year-old men, or 21-year-old men and men with body mass index (BMI) 28, respectively.

There was a strong negative correlation *between* body fat percentage from water weight measurements of eight elderly people *and* daily growth hormone (GH) secretion rate and growth hormone (GH) secretion burst wave amplitude (each r = -0.75 and r = -0.79).

Age and body mass index (BMI) jointly had a significant negative relationship on growth hormone (GH) secretion burst frequency, growth hormone (GH) half-life, mass of growth hormone (GH) secreted per burst, and daily growth hormone (GH) secretion rate. The correlation coefficient for the combined effects of age and body mass index (BMI) on these growth hormone (GH) secretion and systemic clearance parameters was in the range of -0.57 (growth hormone (GH) amount secreted per burst wave) to -0.80 (growth hormone (GH) secretory burst frequency). Therefore, measurement variability and approximately 28-64% clearance of growth hormone (GH) secretion in healthy men is due to the dual effects of age and body mass index (BMI).

Plasma insulin and serum estradiol concentrations were not significant covariates of growth hormone (GH) secretion or clearance in this male cohort. However, there were some positive relationship between plasma somatomedin-C with insulin-like growth factor (IGF-I) and (total or free) testosterone concentrations, and measurement of growth hormone (GH) secretion and clearance. Serum testosterone levels decreased with increasing age and body mass index (BMI) (r = -0.52; p = 0.02). Regression analysis revealed that both body mass index (BMI) and testosterone concentration have exhibited the adverse effect (negative effect) of age on growth hormone (GH) secretion burst frequency persists ($p = 0.007$).

This experiment is in contrast to the previous report [7] of men and women, there was no relationship between serum levels of growth hormone (GH) and estradiol. However, the current study was different from the previous research on many points, including the type and sensitivity of the growth hormone (GH) potency test used, the frequency of blood collection, the subject's restriction to men only, and the use of deconvolution analysis [21].

2.2. Melatonin (Nocturnal Hormones)

Melatonin (**1**) (Figure 1) is one of the hormones produced by the small organ *pineal gland* near the center of the brain. It (**1**) helps to regulate the sleep cycle in the human body, and exerts antioxidative effects on reactive oxygen species (ROS).

The *pineal gland* is a neuroendocrine transducer which regulates several season-dependent events such as sexual activity, deer antler replacement, horn growth, molting, *etc* in certain mammals [22]. However, inferences about potential functions of melatonin (**1**) include physiological symptoms such as sexual maturity, circadian rhythm, jet lag, sleep, depression, *etc.* [23]. It is known that melatonin (**1**) secretion in humans has separately circadian secretion patterns of low levels during the day and high levels during the night.

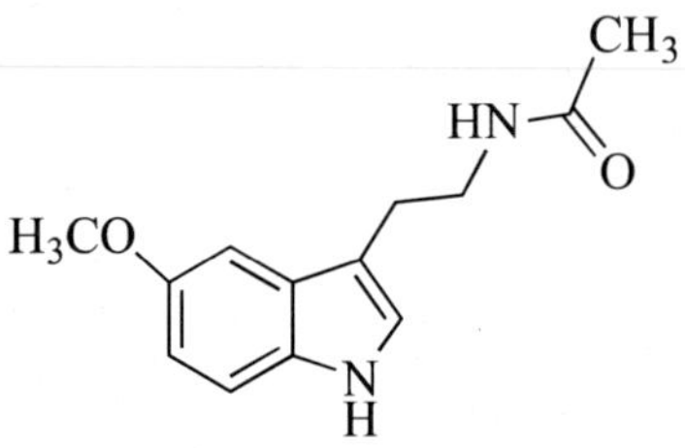

melatonin (**1**)

Figure 1. Melatonin (**1**).

Previous reports [24-28] are not conclusive, however, the potential age-related decline in serum melatonin (**1**) concentrations, especially at night during sexual maturation, is well worth the trouble [29].

Nocturnal serum melatonin (**1**) concentrations in young adults (adolescents between 15 and 30 years of age. adolescent and young adult) are 75% lower when compared to those(nighttime serum melatonin (**1**) concentrations) in children under 5 years old [24]. However, with regard to serum melatonin (**1**) concentrations in the morning (7:30 am-10 am) and at night (11 pm-1 am), the reason for this reduction in nighttime serum melatonin (**1**) concentrations was impossible because the number of subjects (89 children, adolescents and young adults) were too few.

Based on many facts, in 1988, a group of Department of Pediatrics and first Department of Surgery, University of Vienna, Austria examined changes in nocturnal serum melatonin (**1**) concentrations with human growth and aging. Specifically, the main research objectives of serum melatonin (**1**) concentrations reduction are: first, it is to clarify whether there is continuous progression with age, or second, there are specific steps for a decrease related to a specific event such as adrenal gland or adolescence. The third purpose is to provide a reference for nocturnal serum melatonin (**1**) concentrations at different age groups. For this purpose, serum melatonin (**1**) concentrations in serum samples were measured from 367 human subjects (210 male and 157 female) of all ages (from 3 days old to 90 years old).

As a result of the above experiment, first, nocturnal serum melatonin (**1**) concentrations (pg/mL) in 367 subjects (210 males and 157 females) from 3 days to 90 years of age changed dramatically with age as follows: Nocturnal serum melatonin (**1**) concentrations (pg/mL) were low in 3-month-old infants. However, nocturnal serum melatonin (**1**) concentrations (pg/mL) began to increase from 3-6 months after birth. Among these generations, children aged 1-3 years showed the highest nocturnal (nighttime) serum melatonin (**1**) concentrations (pg/mL) (average, 329.5 ± 42 (± SE (standard error)) pg/mL (1.43 ± 0.18 nmol/L)). After that, mean nocturnal serum melatonin (**1**) concentrations (pg/mL) decreased according to the biphasic pattern of both nocturnal serum melatonin (**1**) and age until old age as 29.2 ± 6.1 pg/mL (0.13 ± 0.03 nmol/L) for age 70-90 years.

A rapid and progressive decrease of around 80% nocturnal serum melatonin (**1**) concentrations was noted notably in the period of 1-3 years old to 15-20 years (62.5 ± 9.0 pg/mL (0.27 ± 0.04 nmol/L)). After that, a mild decrease in nocturnal serum melatonin (**1**) was observed. A negative correlation existed between nocturnal serum melatonin (**1**) concentrations and age in the 20-90-years-old period (r = -0.44; p <0.001; y (linear transformation) = 84.8 x e - 0.017x). However, when subjects were divided into 4 age groups (20-35, 35-50, 50-70, and 70-90) and nocturnal serum melatonin (**1**) concentrations were analyzed by analysis of variance (ANOVA), the mean nocturnal serum melatonin (**1**) concentrations revealed a significant difference [F (F statistic) = 28.4; $p < 0.001$)] among the 4 groups. From a *post hoc test* (Tuckey test) which is an inter-group test of multiple comparisons performed after analysis of variance, nocturnal serum melatonin (**1**) concentrations in elderly subjects (70-90 years) showed lower nocturnal serum melatonin (**1**) concentration ($p < 0.01$) when compared to those(nocturnal serum melatonin (**1**) concentrations) in other three group subjects. However, on nocturnal serum melatonin (**1**) concentrations, there was no difference among the three young adult subject groups (20-35, 35-50, and 50-70 years old).

If nocturnal serum melatonin (**1**) concentrations in subjects 1-20 years of age are related to measurements of body size such as height, weight, chest circumference, there was a strong negative relationship between logarithms and body weight of nocturnal serum melatonin (**1**) concentrations (r = -0.54; p < 0.001). A relationship was then drawn between the logarithm of nocturnal serum melatonin (**1**) concentrations and body surface area (r = -0.71; p < 0.001). However, no such relationship was found at age 20-90 (nocturnal serum melatonin (**1**) concentrations, body weight: r = 0.10; p = 0.409; nocturnal serum melatonin (**1**) concentrations *versus* body surface area: r = 0.17; p = 0.224).

There was no relationship between age and daytime serum melatonin (**1**) concentrations. In 59.3% of the subjects, daytime serum melatonin (**1**) concentrations were below the detection limit. In addition, daytime serum melatonin (**1**) concentrations did not differ at night. There was no difference in nocturnal serum melatonin (**1**) concentrations or daytime serum melatonin (**1**) concentrations between men and women [30].

2.3. Thyrotropin (Thyroid-Stimulating Hormone (TSH))

Thyrotropin (TSH. **2**) (Figure 2) is a hormone that is secreted from thyroid stimulating hormone-secreting cells (thyrotrophs) in the anterior pituitary at the base of the brain in response to signals from the hypothalamus of the brain. This thyrotropin (TSH. **2**) then works on the thyroid and stimulates the secretion of two thyroid hormones (thyroxine (T4. **3**) and triiodothyronine (TIT. T3. **4**)) (Figure 2). When thyroid hormones (thyroxine (T4. **3**) and triiodothyronine (TIT. T3. **4**)) are in excess, the anterior pituitary leaves thyrotropin (**2**) production and reduces thyroid hormones (thyroxine (T4. **3**) and triiodothyronine (TIT. T3. **4**)) production. This mechanism maintains the homeostasis of thyroid hormones (thyroxine (T4. **3**) and triiodothyronine (TIT. T3. **4**)) circulating in the blood.

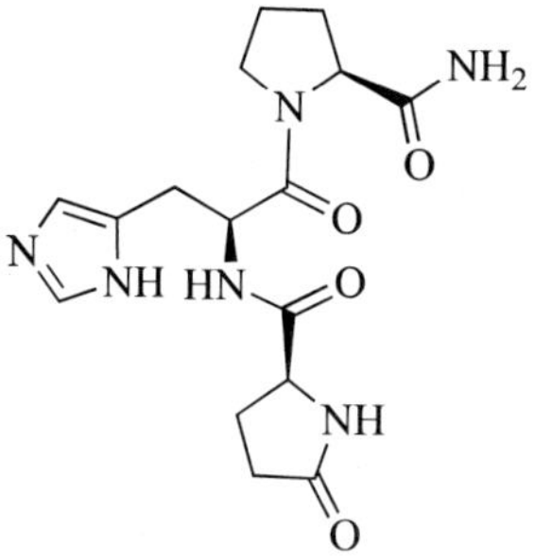

thyrotropin (**2**)

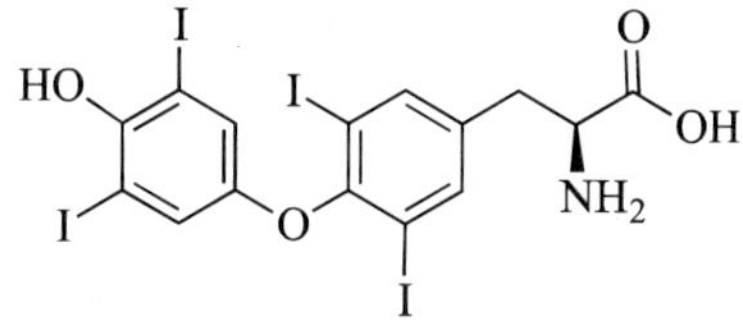

thyroxine (T4. **3**)

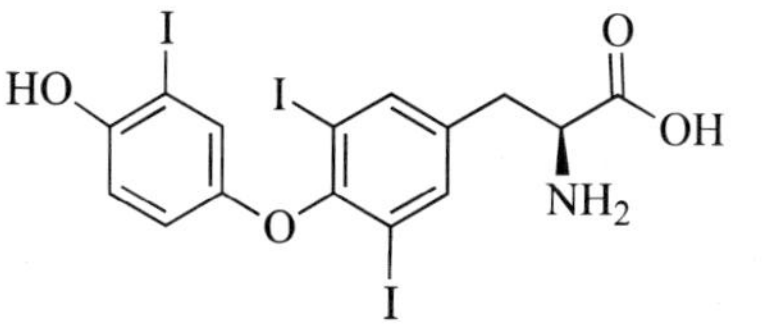

triiodothyronine (TIT. T3. **4**)

Figure 2. Thyrotropin (**2**), and two thyroid hormones (thyroxine (T4. **3**) triiodothyronine (TIT. T3. **4**)).

In 1991, a group of Division of Endocrinology and Metabolism, University of Massachusetts Medical School, Worcester. USA examined the relationship between age, gender, serum thyroxine (T4. **3**) (Figure 2) concentrations and serum thyrotropin (TSH. **2**) concentrations for 202 primary hypothyroid patients in the age range of 10-89.

To predict serum thyrotropin (TSH. **2**) concentrations, multiple linear regression analysis including factors such as age, gender, group, and free serum thyroxine (T4. **3**) index, or free serum thyroxine (T4. **3**) concentration was conducted separately or in combination with the findings from the two male and female patient groups.

As a result, in comparison of all factors, there was negative relationship *between* free serum thyroxine (T4. **3**) index, or free serum thyroxine (T4. **3**) concentration, and age, *and* serum thyrotropin (TSH. **2**) concentrations (p <0.001). In contrast, there was no significant relationship between gender and serum thyrotropin (TSH. **2**) concentrations among these hypothyroid patients. There was a marked relationship *between* hypothyroidism *and* decreased serum thyrotropin (TSH. **2**) concentrations with age in adolescent and adult early (10-39 years) and elderly subjects (61-89). Thus, a decrease in serum thyrotropin (TSH. **2**) concentrations due to age-related hypothyroidism is evident in adolescent and early adult age (10-39 years) and the elderly (61-89 years). These results suggest that age is independent of thyroid concentration and that age is a determinant of thyrotropin (TSH. **2**) secretion [31].

2.4. Thyroid Hormones

Radioimmunoassay (RIA) against two thyroid hormones (thyroxine (T4. **3**) and triiodothyronine (TIT. T3. **4**) has been used for clinical testing. At first, a good relationship has been reported between thyroxine (T4. **3**) and triiodothyronine (TIT. T3. **4**) [32]. However, the *normal range* of each of these two thyroid hormones is quite different. Three main reasons for this are as follows:

First, there is no standard analysis method according to the international standard evaluation method for iodine intake [33, 34].

The second was that thyroxine (T4. **3**) and triiodothyronine (TIT. T3. **4**) concentrations were not normally distributed, but were age-dependent. Furthermore, thyroxine (T4. **3**) showed a more pronounced decrease when compared to that(decrease) of triiodothyronine (TIT. T3. **4**) [35, 36].

Third, serum thyroxine (T4. **3**) and triiodothyronine (TIT. T3. **4**) concentrations from subjects with normal thyroid function (euthyroid subjects) were not always consistent with normal values of both serum thyroxine (T4. **3**) and triiodothyronine (TIT. T3. **4**) concentrations in healthy subjects from other different populations [37].

Based on the above facts, in 1977, a group at Hanover Medical University and Pediatrics, Internal Medicine, Endocrinology, Gottingen, Germany examined that whether serum thyroxine (T4. **3**)-binding globulin (TBG) concentration was partly involved in the large spread of serum thyroxine (T4. **3**) and serum triiodothyronine (TIT. T3. **4**) concentrations *and* their age dependence.

As a result, first, serum thyroxine (T4. **3**)-binding globulin (TBG) clearly showed age-dependent changes as follows:

Cord blood group (number(n):5) was 1.14 ± 0.18 mg TBG/100 mL, and followed by around 1.30 mg TBG/100 mL and 0.14 mean ± standard deviation (SD) for age 1/12-6/12 years old (n = 13) group, around 1.44 mg TBG/100 mL and 0.14 mean ± SD for age 7/12-2 years old (n = 13) group, around 1.30 mg TBG/100 mL and 0.16 mean ± SD for age 5-12 years old (n = 15) group, around 0.95 mg TBG/100 mL and 0.14 mean ± SD for age 19-29 years old (n = 28) group, around 1.08 mg TBG/100 mL and 0.10 mean ± SD for age 30-45 years old (n = 6) group, around 1.28 mg TBG/100 mL and 0.15 mean ± SD for age 60-95 years old (n = 6) group, respectively.

In the one-month age group until puberty, their plasma contained high concentrations of serum thyroxine (T4. **3**)-binding globulin (TBG). These serum thyroxine (T4. **3**)-binding globulin (TBG) concentrations were significantly elevated when compared to the average of 0.98 ± 0.14 mg TBG/100 mL in the middle aged (19-45 years) which usually points to the "*normal range*".

Second, on the course of serum thyroxine (T4. **3**) and triiodothyronine (TIT. T3. **4**) concentrations from birth to old age, both serum thyroxine (T4. **3**) and triiodothyronine (TIT. T3. **4**) concentrations increase sharply during the first 3 hours of birth and reached a stable concentration (plateau) within a week and maintained until adolescence. The plateau concentrations are 10.25 ± 1.62 μg/I00 mL for serum thyroxine (T4. **3**) and 1.62 ± 0.35 ng/mL for serum triiodothyronine (TIT. T3. **4**), respectively.

Regarding two serum thyroxine (T4. **3**) and serum triiodothyronine (TIT. T3. **4**) concentrations, these two mean concentrations in the adolescent group showed a significantly higher concentration ($p < 0.01$) when compared to two mean concentrations in the middle-aged group, i.e., 7.27 ± 2.26 μg/100 mL for serum thyroxine (T4. **3**) and 1.15 ± 0.24 ng/mL for serum triiodothyronine (TIT. T3. **4**), respectively. Two mean concentrations at puberty group is 8.74 ± 2.27 μg/l00 mL for serum thyroxine (T4. **3**) and 1.36 ± 0.36 ng/mL for serum triiodothyronine (TIT. T3. **4**), respectively.

Third, regarding reduction of serum thyroid hormone (serum thyroxine (T4. **3**) and serum triiodothyronine (TIT. T3. **4**) amounts in two age groups, serum thyroid hormone levels in the old age group showed a marked decrease of 21% for serum thyroxine (T4. **3**) and 32% for serum triiodothyronine (TIT. T3. **4**) when compared to those(decreases) of the middle age group.

In general, thyroid hormone binds to serum thyroxine (T4. **3**)-binding globulin (TBG), thyroxine-bound prealbumin thyroxine-binding prealbumin (TBPA), and human serum albumin (HSA). Serum thyroxine (T4. **3**)-binding globulin (TBG) is the protein with the highest binding affinity for both serum thyroxine (T4. **3**) and serum triiodothyronine (TIT. T3. **4**). Thus, serum thyroxine (T4. **3**)-binding globulin (TBG) is known to significantly affect the concentration of each of these two thyroid hormones.

From the above experimental results, *first*, the age-related changes in thyroid hormone, except for the old age, could be explained as being age-dependent by serum thyroxine (T4. **3**)-binding globulin (TBG) concentrations.

Second, it was understood that serum thyroxine (T4. **3**) concentration and serum triiodothyronine (TIT. T3. **4**) concentration in the old age showed a deviation from what expected by their serum thyroxine (T4. **3**)-binding globulin (TBG) concentration.

Third, it suggests that the thyroid hormone/serum thyroxine (T4. **3**)-binding globulin (TBG) ratio is to be possible importance of daily use for early detection in the diagnosis of thyroid diseases such as hypothyroidism where thyroid hormone secretion is abnormal or inflammation occurs [38].

2.5. Calcitonin (CT)

Calcitonin (CT. **5**) is a thyroid peptide hormone that is secreted from the parafollicular cells (or C cells (abbreviated to calcitonin cells)) of the thyroid in mammals. Calcitonin (CT. **5**) is mainly responsible for blood calcium lowering.

Several radioimmunoassays (RIAs) have been used to measure plasma calcitonin (CT. **5**) in humans. However, the determination of plasma calcitonin (CT. **5**) hormone is very difficult due to two reasons: its low basal circulating concentration in plasma and its molecular heterogeneity [39]. Fortunately, a novel sensitive direct radioimmunoassay suitable for plasma calcitonin (CT. **5**) measurement of small samples such as less than 3 pg/mL calcitonin (CT. **5**) is reported, recently.

In 1988, a research group of the Medical Clinics, University of Parma, Parma, Italy set plasma calcitonin (CT. **5**) reference range in normal women using this sensitive direct radioimmunoassay, and evaluated the relationship between plasma calcitonin (CT. **5**) and age.

As a result, first, the values of biochemical limiting factors (parameters) of 67 female healthy subjects were as follows:

Calcium (Ca mg/dL): 9.1 (mean value. mean) ± 0.47 (standard deviation. SD); phosphoric acid (phosphate mg/dL): 3.4 (mean) ± 0.71 (SD); alkaline phosphatase (ALP U/L): 106 (mean) ± 28.9 (SD); calcitonin (CT. **5**) (CT pg/mL): 7.4 (mean) ± 3.1 (SD); parathyroid hormone (parathormone. PTH) (pg/mL): 178 (mean) ± 69.4 (SD).

Second, calcitonin (CT. **5**) concentration was distributed with positive skewness and positive kurtosis. Thus, the reference range for calcitonin (CT. **5**) concentration was derived using both the 2.5^{th} and 97.5^{th} percentile nonparametric tests. As a result, the range limit of calcitonin (CT. **5**) concentration was 3.6-16.9 pg/mL. There were no statistically significant differences for each age group of calcitonin (CT. **5**) concentration among the four age female groups (20-34, 35-50, 51-65, 66-80 years) ($F = 1.7$; $p > 0.05$). Plasma calcitonin (CT. **5**) concentrations were not affected, especially during the 15 years before and after menopause. Plasma calcitonin (CT. **5**) concentrations in a subset of women (20-60 years, mean + SD = 40.4 ± 12.3) showed a significantly lower value when compared to those (plasma calcitonin (CT. **5**) concentrations) in 27 normal male groups at the same age (7.7 ± 2.97 (female) *vs* 11.9 ± 3.97 (male) pg/mL, $F = 23.83$; $p < 0.0001$).

Third, a weak negative relationship was found between plasma calcitonin (CT. **5**) concentrations and age ($r = -0.24$; $p = 0.05$). On the other hand, both parathyroid hormone (PTH) and PTH/CT ratio (parathyroid hormone (PTH)/calcitonin (CT. **5**) ratio) were strongly associated with aging (respectively, $r = 0.43$; $p = 0.0002$; $r = 0.53$; $p < 0.0001$).

From the above results, *first of all*, this novel sensitive direct radioimmunoassay showed sufficient sensitivity to directly evaluate calcitonin (CT. **5**) in a small amount of serum samples of human subjects. *Second*, the novel highly sensitive direct radioimmunoassay gave results similar to those obtained with extraction and purification techniques aimed at measuring calcitonin (CT. **5**) monomers. Therefore, this method is proposed as a new sensitive direct radioimmunoassay for the assay of calcitonin (CT. **5**) assay [40].

2.6. Dehydroepiandrosterone (DHEA)

Dehydroepiandrosterone (DHEA. **7**) (Figure 3) and its sulfated conjugate dehydroepiandrosterone sulfate (DS. DHEAS. **6**) are steroid hormones produced mainly by the adrenal gland. In humans, these two steroid hormones (**6** and **7**) circulate at high concentrations in blood vessels. These steroid hormones (**6** and **7**) are precursors for extra-adrenal synthesis of androgen (**8**) (Figure 3), also called male sex hormone, and estrogen (**9**) (Figure 3), also called female hormone [41]. The functional activities of these two types of steroid hormones (**6** and **7**) have antioxidant properties, suppression of weight gain, suppression of cell proliferation, cancer protection promotion, *etc.* [42, 43, 44].

In 1984, a group at Orentreich Foundation for the Advancement of Science, New York, USA examined age-related changes and gender differences on serum dehydroepiandrosterone sulfate (DS. **6**) concentrations by cross-sectional survey using 981 males and 481 females aged 11 to 89 years. The analysis results from this cross-sectional survey was distributed asymmetrically and normalized by logarithmic transformation. Subsequently, subject groups were analyzed by grouping every 5 years such as 15-19 years old, 20-24 years old, *etc.*

1. male hormones (androgen. **8***)*

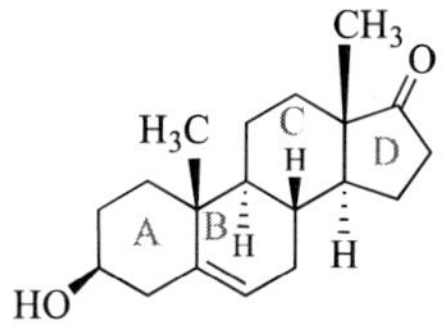

dehydroepiandrosterone (DHEA. 7)

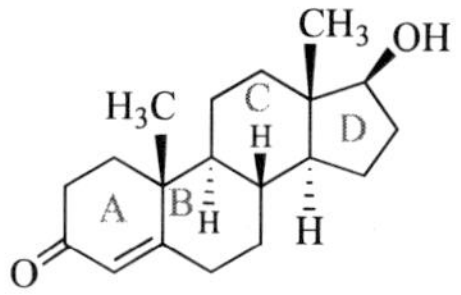

testosterone (**8.1**)

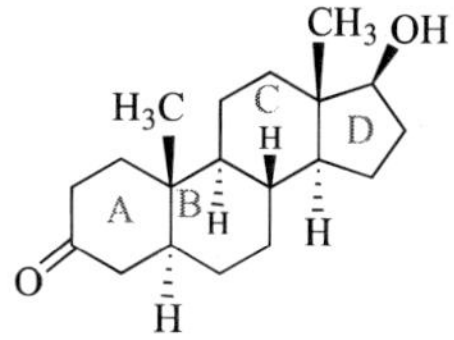

dihydrotestosterone (DHT. **8.2**)

2. female hormones (estrogen. **9***)*

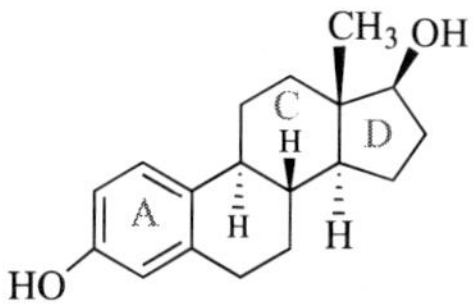

estradiol (**9.1**)

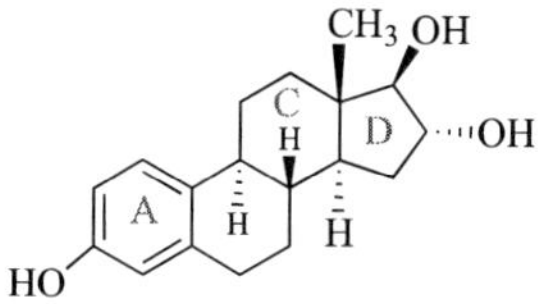

estriol (**9.2**)

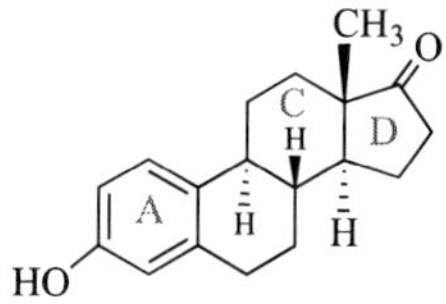

estrone (**9.3**)

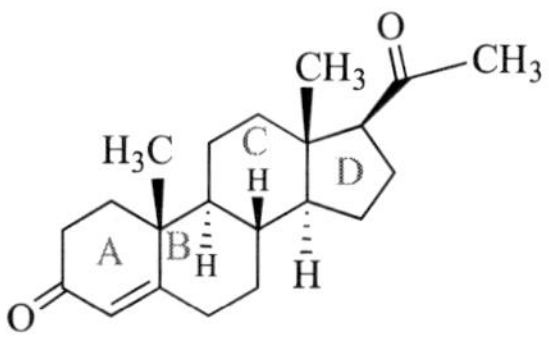

progesterone (**9.4**)

Figure 3. Sex hormones: 1. Male hormones (androgen. **8**) [dehydroepiandreosterone (DHEA. **7**), testesterone (**8.1**), dihydrotestesterone (DHT. **8.2**)], and 2. Female hormones (estrogen. **9**) [estradiol (**9.1**), estriol (**9.2**), estrone (**9.3**) and a gestagen progesterone (**9.4**)].

As a result, first, among subject age group every 5 years, serum dehydroepiandrosterone sulfate (DS. **6**) concentrations reached the highest value in 20-24 year-old group for men (log average, 3470 ng/mL), and 15-19 year-old group for women (log average, 2470 ng/mL). After that, the mean value of serum dehydroepiandrosterone sulfate (DS. **6**) concentrations decreased steadily in both men and women. Regarding the logarithmic average of serum dehydroepiandrosterone sulfate (DS. **6**) concentrations in men and women of aged 70 and over, the 670 ng/mL for men showed a significantly higher value when compared to 450 ng/mL for women. In addition, in terms of the log mean of the 20-69-year-old group, the men group showed a significantly higher value when compared to the women group.

Second, regarding 517 female subjects sera that were frozen and stored for 10-15 years, the random sampling method gave results that were indistinguishable from the values obtained from fresh serum samples. In a supplementary study, longitudinal analysis (longitudinal modal analysis) on weekly fresh serum samples from 4 healthy males aged 36-59 indicated that there were distinct individual differences (average coefficient of variation, 19%). In addition, longitudinal analysis (longitudinal modal analysis) did not show monthly, seasonal, or yearly periodic change. Based on the above analysis results, it is suggested that the normal serum dehydroepiandrosterone sulfate (DS. **6**) concentrations range for adult men and women might be one clinical reference as serum dehydro-epiandrosterone sulfate (DS. **6**) concentrations range in each age group [45].

Aging has been considered as one of the greatest risk factors that cause cancer, dementia, arteriosclerosis, osteoporosis, diabetes, renal failure and heart failure. The major circulating adrenal hormone dehydro-epiandrosterone sulfate (DS. DHEAS. **6**) has been suggested to be involved in many such age-related diseases and possibly aging itself even. However, till now, there is no epidemiological record of dehydro-epiandrosterone sulfate (DS. DHEAS. **6**) in normal adults in Korea. Therefore, in 1998, a group at the Department of Family Medicine, Pochon Jung Moon Medical University, Korea has examined age changes and sex differences in serum dehydroepiandrosterone sulfate (DS. DHEAS. **6**) and its related factors throughout adulthood.

First, regarding the survey method, questionnaires were prepared for all subjects. Serum dehydroepiandrosterone sulfate (DS. DHEAS. **6**) concentration, and biochemical markers such as total cholesterol, triglycerides, high-density lipoprotein cholesterol (HDL cholesterol), glucose in 1710 healthy adults aged 17-76 (857 males and 853 females) were measured. Furthermore, the height, weight, waist (hip circumference), and body fat mass in subjects were indirectly determined by the bioimpedance method using the electrical impedance (electrical resistance of living body used for body fat percentage measurement *etc*) through flowing a weak current into the body. Then, statistical analysis software SPSS was used to analyze various variables related to serum dehydroepiandrosterone sulfate (DS. DHEAS. **6**) concentration. At the same time, reference data of serum dehydroepiandrosterone sulfate (DS. DHEAS. **6**) concentration in normal adults were also presented.

Second, regarding the average serum dehydroepiandrosterone sulfate (DS. DHEAS. **6**) concentration (μg/dL) by gender age group of men and women, the change rate (%) by comparison of average serum dehydroepiandrosterone sulfate (DS. DHEAS. **6**) concentration (μg/dL) less than 30 years old with average serum dehydroepiandrosterone sulfate (DS. DHEAS. **6**) concentration (μg/dL) over 30 years old was as follows:

Serum dehydroepiandrosterone sulfate (DS. DHEAS. **6**) concentration (μg/dL), and percent change (%) in men were 260.9 (mean) ± 87.74 (standard deviation. SD), 100% for men younger than 30 years (number of subjects n = 25); 259.0 (mean) ± 128.90 (SD), 99.3% for men aged 30-34 (n = 100); 241.4 (mean) ± 117.81 (SD), 92.5% for men aged 35-39 (n = 175); 227.0 (mean value) ± 108.53 (SD), 87.0% for men aged 40-44 (n = 203); 213.9 (mean) ± 100.02 (SD), 82.0% for men aged 45-49 (n = 111); 188.8 (mean value) ± 121.74 (SD), 72.4% for men aged 50-54 (n = 82); 143.7 (mean) ± 78.87 (SD), 55.1% for men aged 55-59 (n = 82); 123.4 (mean) ± 84.63 (SD), 47.3% for men aged 60-64 (n = 51); 94.0 (mean value) ± 43.47 (SD), 36.0% for men aged 65-69 (n = 15); 80.7 (mean value) ± 34.28 (SD), 30.9% for men aged 70 and over (n = 9), respectively.

Serum dehydroepiandrosterone sulfate (DS. DHEAS. **6**) concentration (μg/dL), and percent change (%) in women were 203.6 (mean value) ± 124.15 (SD), 100% for women under the age of 30 (number of subjects n = 60), 188.1 (mean value) ± 104.06 (SD), 92.4% for women aged 30-34 (n = 114); 160.6 (mean value) ± 112.12 (SD), 78.9% for women aged 35-39 (n = 179); 141.6 (mean) ± 79.20 (SD), 69.5% for women aged 40-44 (n = 137); 123.8 (mean value) ± 77.64 (SD), 60.8% for women aged 45-49 (n = 88); 106.3 (mean) ± 79.29 (SD), 52.2% for women aged 50-54 (n = 94); 73.3 (mean value) ± 42.87 (SD), 36.0% for women aged 55-59 (n = 72);

61.8 (mean value) ± 47.36 (SD), 30.4% for women aged 60-64 (n = 65); 57.5 (mean value) ± 36.77 (SD), 28.2% for women aged 65-69 (n = 28); 61.8 (mean value) ± 41.00 (SD), 30.4% for women over 70 (n = 20), respectively.

From the above results, first, in men, peak of serum dehydro-epiandrosterone sulfate (DS. DHEAS. **6**) concentration (μg/dL) reached in the age group less than 30 years (260.9 (mean) ± 87.74 (SD), change rate 100%). Similarly, in women, peak of serum dehydro-epiandrosterone sulfate (DS. DHEAS. **6**) concentration (μg/dL) reached in the age group less than 30 years (203.6 (mean) ± 124.15 (SD), change rate 100%). After that, mean values decreased steadily with age for both men and women ($r = -0.38$, $p < 0.001$ for men; $r = -0.46$, $p < 0.001$ for women).

Second, when serum dehydroepiandrosterone sulfate (DS. DHEAS. **6**) concentration (μg/dL) in age group over 70 years old compared to serum dehydroepiandrosterone sulfate (DS. DHEAS. **6**) concentration (μg/dL) in age group less than 30 years old, only 30.9% remained in men and 30.4% in women.

In all age groups except age group 70 years or older, serum dehydroepiandrosterone sulfate (DS. DHEAS. **6**) concentration (μg/dL) in men was significantly higher than that(serum DHEAS (**6**)) in women. Serum dehydroepiandrosterone sulfate (DS. DHEAS. **6**) concentration (μg/dL) of each male age group was an average 1.5 times higher than that(serum DHEAS (**6**)) of the corresponding female age group. Males under 30 years of age show at least 1.28 times higher concentrations than those(serum DHEAS (**6**)) of females and 60-64 years old males show concentrations up to 2.00 times higher than that(serum DHEAS (**6**)) of females.

Third, age-adjusted mean standard error (SE) serum dehydro-epiandrosterone sulfate (DS. DHEAS. **6**) concentration (μg/dL) by risk factor categories for men and women is as follows:

First, for smoking, male smokers (n = 521): 218.1 (mean) ± 4.7 (SE) ($p = 0.016$); female smokers (n = 47): 121.2 (mean value) ± 13.2 (SE)($p = 0.262$), and male non smoker (n = 297): 199.1 (mean value) ± 6.3 (SE); female non smoker (n = 623): 136.6 (mean value) ± 3.6 (SE).

Second, for drinking (more than twice a week), male drinkers (n = 638): 219.1 (mean) ± 4.2 (SE) ($p = 0.001$); female drinkers (n = 86): 154.3 (mean) ± 9.6 (SE) ($p = 0.026$), and male non-drinkers (n = 188): 185.3 (mean) ± 7.8 (SE); female non-drinkers (n = 698): 131.7 (mean value) ± 3.4 (SE).

Third, for exercise (more than 3 times a week), male activists(n = 233): 215.9 (mean value) ± 7.1 (SE) ($p = 0.045$); female activists (n = 196): 146.1 (mean value) ± 6.4 (SE) ($p = 0.051$), and male non-exercisers (n = 579): 209.5 (mean value) ± 4.5 (SE); female non-exerciser (n = 598): 131.6 (mean value) ± 3.7 (SE).

Fourth, for obesity: regarding obesity (body mass index (BMI): less than 20), male obese (n = 80): 187.4 (mean) ± 12.0 (SE) ($p = 0.039$), and female obesc (n = 168): 135.6 (mean) ± 2.1 (SE) ($p = 0.966$).

For obesity (body mass index (BMI): 20 or more and less than 27), male obese (n = 675): 211.6 (mean value) ± 4.1 (SE), and female obese (n = 586): 133.5 (mean value) ± 3.7 (SE).

For obesity (body mass index (BMI): 27 or more), male obese (n = 98): 228.2 (mean value) ± 10.8 (SE), and female obese (n = 103): 133.9 (mean value) ± 8.9 (SE),

Fifth, body fat distribution: With respect to the female type (gynecoid type) of body fat distribution, male obese (n = 519): 197.4 (mean value) ± 4.6 (SE) ($p = 0.001$), and female obese (n = 534): 131.5 (mean value) ± 4.1 (SE) ($p = 0.278$).

Regarding the male type (android type) of body fat distribution, male obese (n = 288): 227.1 (mean value) ± 6.2 (SE), and female obese (n = 290): 139.8 (mean value) ± 5.8 (SE).

Sixth, hypertension: regarding less than stage 2 hypertension, male hypertensive (n = 786): 211.6 (mean) ± 3.8 (SE) ($p = 0.725$), and female hypertensive (n = 793): 133.8 (mean) ± 3.1 (SE) ($p = 0.846$).

For stage 2 or higher hypertension, male hypertensive (n = 67): 206.7 (mean) ± 13.4 (SE), and female hypertensive person (n = 64): 136.1 (mean value) ± 11.3 (SE).

Seventh, serum total cholesterol (total cholesterol): for total cholesterol less than 240 mg/dL,_male subjects (n = 761): 210.5 (mean value) ± 3.9

(SE) (p = 0.557), and female subject (n = 754): 133.0 (mean value) ± 3.2 (SE) ($p = 0.368$).

For total cholesterol 240 mg/dL or more, male subject (n = 92): 217.5 (mean value) ± 11.2 (SE), and female subject (n = 103): 141.5 (mean value) ± 8.9 (SE).

Eighth, serum triglyceride (neutral fat): For less than 250 mg/dL neutral fat, male subjects (n = 725): 209.0 (mean value) ± 4.0 (SE)(p = 0.148), and female subject (n = 800): 134.5 (mean value) ± 3.1 (SE)(p = 0.512).

For neutral fat 250 mg/L or more, male subject (n = 128): 223.9 (mean value) ± 9.5 (SE), and female subject (n = 57): 127.2 (mean value) ± 12.1 (SE).

Ninth, serum high density lipoprotein cholesterol (HDL cholesterol): Regarding HDL cholesterol less than 35 mg/dL, male subjects (n = 120): 212.9 (mean) ± 9.9 (SE) ($p = 0.826$), and female subject (n = 34): 136.3 (mean value) ± 15.3 (SE) ($p = 0.902$).

For HDL cholesterol 35 mg/dL or higher, male subject (n = 697): 210.6 (mean value) ± 4.1 (SE), and female subject (n = 812): 134.4 (mean value) ± 3.1 (SE).

Tenth, serum low density lipoprotein cholesterol (LDL cholesterol): Regarding LDL cholesterol less than 160 mg/dL, male subjects (n = 780): 212.2 (mean value) ± 9.9 (SE) ($p = 0.404$), and female subjects (n = 766): 133.0 (mean value) ± 3.2 (SE) ($p = 0.364$).

For LDL cholesterol 160 mg/dL or more, male subjects (n = 73): 201.2 (mean value) ± 12.6 (SE), and female subject (n = 91): 142.1 (mean value) ± 9.5 (SE).

Eleventh, blood sugar: For blood sugar less than 126 mg/dL, male subject (n = 812): 211.8 (mean) ± 3.8 (SE) ($p = 0.469$), and female subject (n = 833): 134.1 (mean value) ± 3.1 (SE) ($p = 0.895$).

As for blood sugar 126 mg/L or more, male subject (n = 41): 199.9 (mean value) ± 17.0 (SE), and female subject (n = 24): 131.6 (mean value) ± 8.2 (SE).

Twelve, menopause: menopausal female subjects (n = 268): 127.6 (mean value) ± 7.4 (SE) (p = 0.152). Non-menopausal female subjects (n = 491): 142.3 (mean value) ± 4.9 (SE).

From the above *1-12* results, in men, serum dehydroepiandrosterone sulfate (DS. DHEAS. **6**) concentration (μg/dL) showed higher value when their mean values of smokers (218.1(smokers) *vs.* 199.1(non-smokers) μg/dL, $p < 0.05$), drinkers (2 or more/week, 219.1(drinkers) *vs* 185.3(non-drinkers) μg/dL, $p < 0.01$), android type fat distribution group (waist/hip > 0.85, 227.1(male type) *vs* 197.4(female type) μg/dL μg/dL) were compared to (DS (DHEAS. **6**)) of mean non-smoker, non-drinker or female type fat distribution group.

There was a positive relationship between serum dehydro-epiandrosterone sulfate (DS. DHEAS. **6**) concentration (μg/dL) and body mass index (BMI) ($r = 0.12$, $p < 0.01$).

However, in women, the mean of serum dehydroepiandrosterone sulfate (DS. DHEAS. **6**) concentration (μg/dL) on the drinker (154.3 (drinker) *vs* 131.7(non-drinker) μg/dL, $p < 0.05$) and the regular exercise group (146.1(exerciser) *vs* 131.6(non-exercise) μg/dL, $p = 0.05$) was higher when compared to that (DS (DHEAS. **6**)) of non-drinker, or non-exercise.

There was no significant relationship between serum dehydro-epiandrosterone sulfate (DS. DHEAS. **6**) concentration (μg/dL), lipid profile (total cholesterol, triglyceride, HDL cholesterol, LDL cholesterol), and fasting glucose level in both men and women.

From results of First - Third above, it is suggested that serum dehydroepiandrosterone sulfate (DS. DHEAS. **6**) concentration (μg/dL) is influenced by several sociodemographic factors such as smoking, alcohol, exercise and body mass index (BMI). There is a negative relationship between serum dehydroepiandrosterone sulfate (DS. DHEAS. **6**) concentration (μg/dL) and age in both men and women, males showed approximately 1.5 times higher serum dehydroepiandrosterone sulfate (DS. DHEAS. **6**) concentration (μg/dL) than females. Furthermore, there was no association between serum dehydroepiandrosterone sulfate (DS. DHEAS. **6**) concentration (μg/dL) and lipid profile and fasting blood glucose [46].

2.7. Aldosterone

Aldosterone (**10**) (Figure 4) is a type of mineralocorticoid hormone produced by adrenal cortex. Aldosterone (**10**) is a corticosteroid that regulates sodium reabsorption.

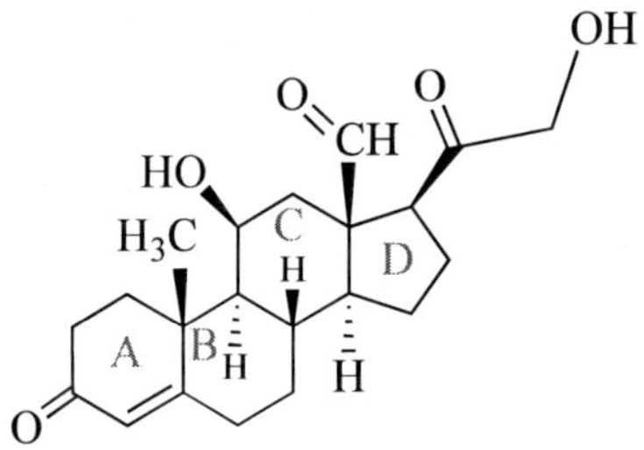
aldosterone (**10**)

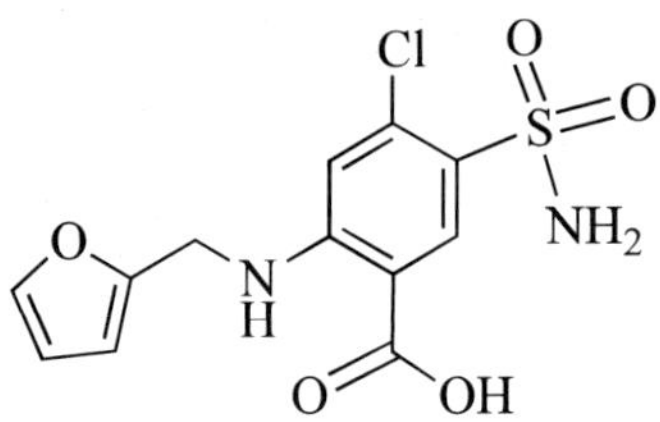
furosemide (**11**)

Figure 4. Aldosterone (**10**) and furosemide (**11**).

In 1983, a group of University of Oklahoma College of Medicine, Oklahoma City, Oklahoma USA measured the amount of urinary aldosterone (**10**) and plasma aldosterone (**10**) in healthy subjects aged 20-59 years during the period of an unlimited sodium intake and after period of sodium deficiency, using a loop diuretic furosemide (**11**) (Figure 4) or a 20 meq (milli equivalent) sodium equivalent diet.

Here, aldosterone (**10**) is a kind of mineralocorticoid hormone among steroid hormones secreted from adrenal cortex (outer layer of adrenal gland). Aldosterone (**10**) has the effect of removing potassium outside the body while retaining sodium in the body. So, aldosterone (**10**) is involved in balancing the water and salt in the kidney. On the other hand, excessive aldosterone (**10**) in the body may cause an increase in blood pressure and retention of fluid in body tissues.

In addition, loop diuretic inhibits the movement of water in the henreloop in the kidney tubule, thereby has a function for reducing the amount of water in the body and excreting the water out of the body as urine.

As a result, first, regarding before and after sodium deficiency, the average and upper limits of urinary aldosterone (**10**) excretion range for subjects under 30 years of age are significantly higher when compared to those(the mean and upper limits of urinary aldosterone (**10**) excretion range) of over 50 years of age. Aging did not affect plasma aldosterone (**10**) levels when subjects had uncontrolled sodium intake. At this time, blood was collected while the subjects were lying down.

In contrast to this,_when the subjects were upright both before and after sodium deficiency, the mean and upper limit of the range of plasma aldosterone (**10**) levels in subjects over 50 showed lower values when compared to those(mean and upper limit of the range of plasma **10** levels) for subjects under 30 years of age.

There was no significant difference in plasma aldosterone (**10**) levels metabolic clearance between the young and the elderly.

If the normal range of *recumbency* plasma aldosterone (**10**) levels is not age-adjusted, four of eight patients over the age of 40 with aldosterone (**10**)-producing adenomas showed normal excretion rates of plasma aldosterone (**10**). However, with age adjustment of the plasma aldosterone (**10**) excretion rate, all patients showed clearly high excretion rates.

Similarly, if the normal range of *upright* plasma aldosterone (**10**) levels are not age-adjusted, six out of seven patients over the age of 40 show normal plasma aldosterone (**10**) concentrations.

The above results suggest that plasma aldosterone (**10**) secretion decreases with age regardless of gender.

Approximately 5-10% of hypertensive patients are widely recognized from young people to the elderly is considered that secondary hypertension due to primary aldosteronism (PA) caused by oversecretion of aldosterone (**10**) from adrenal gland becomes the cause [47].

Primary aldosteronism (PA) develops hypertension at a relatively young age caused by hyperplasia, adenomas, or cancer, *etc*., it can cause serious complications such as cerebral hemorrhage besides paroxysmal muscle weakness, elevated blood pressure, and hypokalemia. For the diagnosis of primary hyperaldosteronism (PA), measurements of plasma aldosterone (**10**) level and plasma renin activity (PRA) are performed.

It suggests that the effect of age on plasma aldosterone (**10**) secretion can be an essential consideration in especially diagnosing elderly hypertensive patients in regards to primary hyperaldosteronism (PA) [48].

Both aging and inadequate aldosterone (**10**) secretion are known to increase the risk of developing cardiovascular disease (CVD). However, the relationship between decreased aldosterone (**10**) secretion due to aging and its effect on physiological functions is not well known.

Therefore, in 2017, Departments of Molecular and Integrative Physiology & Internal Medicine, University of Michigan, USA) investigated the relationship between aging and aldosterone (**10**) secretion in age-related autonomous aldosteronism.

Aldosterone (**10**)-producing cell clusters (APCCs) invade the zona fasciculata of the adrenal cortex, have somatic mutations known to increase aldosterone (**10**) secretion. Aldosterone (**10**)-producing cell clusters (APCCs) appear to initiate aldosterone (**10**) secretion, renin-independent and angiotensin II (Ang II)-independent. In this regard, it is believed that aldosterone (**10**)-producing cell clusters (APCCs) are currently the source of the secretion of previously unknown autonomous aldosterone (**10**), and is a potential precursor or attenuated form for the treatment of primary aldosteronism (PA) [49].

As a result, first, regarding the relationship between cytochrome P450 aldosterone synthase (CYP11B2 protein) expression pattern and age in normal adrenal gland by imaging analysis of immunohistochemistry measurement for a total of 127 humans normal adrenal glands ranging from 9 months to 68 years of age, the typical CYP11B2 protein expression pattern of the young *vs.* elderly adrenals was as follows. *First,* continuous CYP11B2 protein expression in the zona glomerulosa (ZG) was more frequently seen in the adrenals of the young than in the adrenals of the elderly. CYP11B2 protein expression of many elderly adrenals showed discrete or did not show glomerular zone (zona glomerulosa. ZG) CYP11B2 protein expression.

Second, from the image analysis results, there was a negative relationship between the total CYP11B2 protein expression area normalized to the adrenal cortex and the age (r = -0.431, p < 0.0001).

There was also a negative relationship between the normal glomerular zone (zona glomerulosa. ZG) calculated by subtracting aldosterone (**10**)-producing cell clusters (APCCs) region from the total CYP11B2 protein expression area and age (normalized to adrenal cortex, r = -0.495, $p < 0.0001$). However, the sum of aldosterone (**10**)-producing cell clusters (APCCs) area normalized to the adrenal cortex showed a positive relationship with age ($r = 0.390$, $p < 0.0001$).

The integral ratio of aldosterone (**10**)-producing cell clusters (APCCs) area to total CYP11B2 protein expression area also showed a positive relationship with age ($r = 0.587$, $p < 0.0001$). The positive relationship between the integral ratio of aldosterone (**10**)-producing cell clusters (APCCs) area to the total CYP11B2 protein expression area and the age apparently suggests a transition *from* the zona glomerulosa (ZG) CYP11B2 protein expression dominance in young people *to* aldosterone (**10**)-producing cell clusters (APCCs) dominant in the elderly.

The relationship between age and the integral ratio of aldosterone (**10**)-producing cell clusters (APCCs) area to total CYP11B2 protein expression area remained significant after adjustment for gender and race ($\beta = + 0.589$, $p < 0.001$).

Third, regarding comparison of CYP11B2 protein expression patterns *between* adrenal glands with aldosterone (**10**)-producing cell clusters (APCCs) *and* adrenal glands without aldosterone (**10**)-producing cell clusters (APCCs), as expected from the donor age, comparing the adrenals of donor-ageers with aldosterone (**10**)-producing cell clusters (APCCs) with adrenals of donor-ageers without aldosterone (**10**)-producing cell clusters (APCCs), adrenals of donor-ageers with at least one aldosterone (**10**)-producing cell clusters (APCCs) were significantly elder donor-ageers ($p < 0.001$). The morbidity rate of continuous zona glomerulosa (ZG) CYP11B2 protein expression region, total CYP11B2 protein expression region normalized to adrenal cortex, and normal zona glomerulosa (ZG) CYP11B2 protein expression region normalized to adrenal cortex in adrenals of donor-ageers with aldosterone (**10**)-producing cell clusters (APCCs) was significantly lower when compred to that(morbidity rate) of adrenals of donor-ageers without aldosterone (**10**)-producing cell clusters (APCCs) ($p < 0.001$, $p = 0.049$, and $p < 0.001$, respectively).

Second, regarding kinetics of aldosterone (**10**) dysregulation and age for 18-71 years old (mean age 44.7 years) clinical subjects in almost white men, *first*, there was an inverse relationship between age and serum panel-reactive antibody (PRA) (β = -0.075 ng/mL per hour every 10 years, $p < 0.01$).

However, even if panel-reactive antibody (PRA) decreases with age, serum aldosterone (**10**) (β = −0.14 ng/L aldosterone (**10**) per 10 years, $p = 0.24$) and 24 hours urinary aldosterone (**10**) excretion (β = -0.30 μg of aldosterone (**10**) per 24 hours every 10 years, $p = 0.31$) showed no significant change with age.

Similarly, regarding the aldosterone/renin ratio (ARR) from the primary aldosteronism detection screening test for high-risk hypertensive persons, serum aldosterone/renin ratio (ARR) of elderly people was higher in serum aldosterone/renin ratio (ARR) as they became elderly people (β = + 3.88 ng/dL per ng/mLper 10 years, $p = 0.001$). The relationship between age and serum aldosterone/renin ratio (ARR) remains significant even after adjusting for gender, race, body mass index (BMI), blood pressure, hypertension status, and urinary sodium excretion. (β = + 5.54 U per 10 years, $p < 0.001$).

Second, the same subject was sodium limited to measure the renin-angiotensin-aldosterone system stimulation. As a result, from panel-reactive antibody (PRA) measurement, the mean supine serum aldosterone (**10**) increased from 3.07(4.08) ng/mL per hour to 9.2 (13.1) ng/dL per hour.

In relation to this, aging showed blunt stimulation for both panel-reactive antibody (PRA) and aldosterone (**10**) (PRA: β = −0.54 ng/mLxh per 10 years, $p < 0.01$; and aldosterone: $\beta = -4.6$ ng/dL per 10 years, $p < 0.0001$).

Third, taking into account the evidence for *both* unrestrained renin-independent aldosteronism *and* aldosterone impairment in the elderly, these physiological responses were integrated into a single metric, namely sodium modulated aldosterone suppression-to-stimulation index (SASSI).

Using SASSI to capture the full range of dysregulated aldosterone (**10**) physiology, gender, race, body mass index (BMI), mean arterial blood pressure, hypertension status, and urinary sodium excretion (unadjusted $\beta = 0.072$, $p < 0.0001$) has been adjusted. However, even then, there was a positive relationship between the elderly and higher SASSI ($\beta = 0.037$, $p < 0.01$).

From the above results, the process of aging is associated with an increase in the amount of adrenal aldosterone (**10**)-producing cell clusters (APCCs). Therefore, the process of aging may be the cause by the concomitant decrease of physiological cytochrome P450 aldosterone synthetase CYP11B2 (CYP11B2 protein) expression that exists in zona glomerulosa (ZG) of the adrenal cortex with increased amounts of adrenal aldosterone (**10**)-producing cell clusters (APCCs). Furthermore, these age-related histopathological changes suggested the possibility which causes an increase in the secretion of the autonomous aldosterone (**10**) found in renin-independent aldosteronism and an accompanying failure against physiological stimulus of aldosterone (**10**) [50].

2.8. Estrogens

Female hormone (estrogen. **9**) is a generic term for steroid hormones, consisting of three type, estradiol (**9.1**), estriol (**9.2**) and estrone (**9.3**) (Figure 3) with female hormone-like activity.

First, with regard to women, estrogen (**9**) deficiency shows rapid bone loss in the early postmenopausal stage. In addition, estrogen (**9**) deficiency also has been known that estrogen (**9**) deficiency may also be involved in bone loss even late period in the late phase with aging. Bone loss at this late stage is mainly due to increase in serum arathyroid hormone (parathormone. PTH) levels with age, and it was due at least in part to the age-related increase in bone turnover (bone metabolism) [51, 52, 53].

However, estrogen (**9**) therapy for postmenopausal elderly women seems to prevent secondary hyperparathyroidism and the increased bone turnover (bone metabolism) *which is one of the risk factors of bone strength* with aging [53, 54].

This fact led to the following hypothesis: Extraosseous (extraskeletal) effect such as absorption of calcium in intestinal tract [55, 56], calcium treatment of the kidney [57, 58], and possibly direct impact to arathyroid hormone (parathormone. PTH) secretion [59] by estrogen (female hormone. **9**) can be a cause of prevention against both age-related increase in serum arathyroid hormone (parathormone. PTH), and the increased bone turnover with age in postmenopausal women treated with estrogen (female hormone. **9**) [60].

Second with regard to men, serum total testosterone (**8.1**) levels decreased only marginally with age, as men do not have male menopausal disorders equivalent to female menopausal disorders [61, 62, 63]. However, according to the cross-sectional analysis [64, 65], as age, bone mineral density (BMD) decreases significantly.

However, from epidemiological studies, there was no relationship between serum total testosteron (**8.1**) levels and bone mineral density (BMD) [63, 66]. Alternatively, there was even no relationship between serum total testosteron (**8.1**) levels and bone mineral density (BMD) in aging men [67]. Then, the lack of a substantial decrease in serum total testosterone (**8.1**) levels in older men means that testosterone (**8.1**) is not one of the main causes of bone loss in older men.

As in women, female hormone (estrogen. **9**) may play an important role in regulating bone turnover in men. Even in the presence of normal testosterone (**8.1**) and free testosterone (**8.1**) levels, men who have homozygous mutations in the female hormone (estrogen. **9**) receptor gene showed unfused epiphyses (unfused bone end) and marked osteopenia along with the increased bone turnover [68].

Based on above facts, in 1998, first, a group of Endocrine Research Unit, Mayo Clinic, Rochester, Minnesota, USA, has examined the relationship between circulating bioavailable testosterone (**8.1**) and female hormone (estrogen. **9**) levels, and age-related changes for 346 male patients aged 23-90 classified by age group on a population basis. Next, this group assesses age-related changes in serum parathyroid hormone (parathormone. PTH) and change by age of markers of bone turnover in these men, and these estimations are associated with bone mineral density (BMD) and sex steroid hormones. Finally, this group conducted a similar study in a parallel cohort of 304 women to compare these relationships between older men and older women.

First, on age-related changes in bone mineral density (BMD) and serum sex steroids: The correlation coefficients (r) for relationship between the age and bone mineral density (BMD), age and serum sex steroid hormone (SH), age and serum sex hormone-binding globulin (SHBG) concentration, age and serum luteinizing hormone (LH), age and serum follicle-stimulating hormone (FSH) concentration among age-stratified samples of Rochester men and women were as follows.

First, the correlation coefficient (r) between age and bone mineral density (BMD) was as follows:

For males, total body: r = -0.29; change rate from 25 to 85 years (%): -7.7, and *for females*, total body: r = -0.62; change rate from 25 to 85 years (%): -17.6.

For males, lateral spine: r = -0.44; change rate from 25 to 85 years (%): -26.8, and *for females*, lateral spine: r = -0.70; change rate from 25 to 85 years (%): -45.2.

For males, proximal femur: r = -0.36; change rate from 25 to 85 years (%):-15.5, and *for females*, proximal femur: r = -0.62; change rate from 25 to 85 years (%): -29.5.

For males, radius: r = -0.51; change rate from 25 to 85 years (%):-17.8, and *for females*, radius: r = -0.70; change rate from 25 to 85 years (%): -28.4.

Second, the correlation coefficient (r) between age and serum sex steroid hormone (SH) was as follows:

For males, total serum testosterone (T. **8.1**): r = -0.25; change rate from 25 to 85 years (%): -29.5, and *for females*, total serum testosterone (T. **8.1**): r = -0.13; change rate from 25 to 85 years (%): -15.8.

For males, bioavailable serum testosterone. T. **8.1**): r = -0.62; change rate from 25 to 85 years (%): -64.1, and *for females*, bioavailable serum testosterone. T. **8.1**): r = -0.16; change rate from 25 to 85 years (%): -28.4.

For males, total serum estrogen (E_1. **9.3**) + estradiol (E_2. **9.1**)): r = -0.09; change rate from 25 to 85 years (%): -11.5, and *for females*, total serum estrogen (E_1. **9.3**) + estradiol (E_2. **9.1**)): r = -0.49; change rate from 25 to 85 years (%): -81.2.

For males, bioavailable serum estrogen (estrone. E_1. **9.3**) + estradiol (E_2. **9.1**)): r = -0.09; change rate from 25 to 85 years (%): -11.5, and *for females*, bioavailable serum estrogen (estrone. E_1. **9.3**) + estradiol (E_2. **9.1**)): r = -0.49; change rate from 25 to 85 years (%): -81.2.

For males, bioavailable serum testosterone (T. **8.1**)/sex hormone-binding globulin (SHBG) concentration (T/SHBG ratio) (log): r = -0.55; change rate from 25 to 85 years (%): -83.2, and *for females*, T/SHBG ratio (log): r = -0.15; change rate from 25 to 85 years (%): -32,3.

For males, serum estrogen (E) (estrone (E_1. **9.3**) + estradiol (E_2. **9.1**))/sex hormone-binding globulin (SHBG) concentration (E/SHBG ratio) (log): r = -0.46; change rate from 25 to 85 years (%): -69.3, and *for females*, T/SHBG ratio (log): r = -0.53; change rate from 25 to 85 years (%): -81.1.

For males, serum free testosterone (T. **8.1**) (log): r = -0.62; change rate from 25 to 85 years (%): -92.4, and *for females*, serum free testosterone (T. **8.1**) (log): r = -0.16; change rate from 25 to 85 years (%): -33.4.

For males, serum dehydroepiandrosterone (DHEA. **7**): r = -0.68; change rate from 25 to 85 years (%): -83.3, and *for females*, serum dehydroepiandrosterone (DHEA. **7**): r = -0.61; change rate from 25 to 85 years (%): -74.5.

Third, the correlation coefficient (r) between age and serum sex hormone-binding globulin (SHBG) concentration was as follows:

For males, serum sex hormone-binding globulin (SHBG) concentration: r = -0.50; change rate from 25 to 85 years (%): 124.3, and *for females*, SHBG: r = -0.03; change rate from 25 to 85 years (%): -1.4.

Fourth, the correlation coefficient (r) between age and serum luteinizing hormone (LH) concentration was as follows:

For males, serum luteinizing hormone (LH) concentration: r = 0.36; change rate from 25 to 85 years (%): 285.5, and *for females*, erum luteinizing hormone (LH) concentration: r = 0.47; change rate from 25 to 85 years (%): 731.4.

Fifth, the correlation coefficient (r) between age and serum follicle-stimulating hormone (FSH) concentration was as follows:

For males, erum follicle-stimulating hormone (FSH) concentration: r = 0.49; change rate from 25 to 85 years (%): 505.2, and *for females*, erum follicle-stimulating hormone (FSH) concentration: r = 0.84; change rate from 25 to 85 years (%): 1804.9.

From the above results, by the cross-sectional analysis of bone mineral density (BMD) and age in men and women aged 25-85, BMD decreased significantly with age for whole body (total body), lateral spine, proximal femur, and radius (bone of the forearm) in both men and women (original Table 1). The rate of decrease of BMD for whole body (total body), lateral spine, proximal femur, and radius in women showed higher reduction rate when compared to these (reduction rate) in men.

In age-related changes in total serum sex steroid hormone (SH) concentration in men and women ranged from 25 to 85 years old, the decrease in bioavailable serum testosterone (T. **8.1**) is approximately twice to that of total serum testosterone (T. **8.1**) in both men and women, and bioavailable serum testosterone (T. **8.1**) was reduced by approximately 64% and 28% in men and women, respectively.

In men, total serum estrogen (E) (estrone (E_1. **9.3**) + stradiol (E_2. **9.1**)) decreased only slightly (-11.5%) with age. However, bioavailable serum estrogen (E) (estrone (E_1. **9.3**) + estradiol (E_2. **9.1**)) decreased by 47.1%.

In contrast to these men, in women, total serum estrogen (E) (estrone (E_1. **9.3**) + estradiol (E_2, **9.1**)) (-81.2) and bioavailable serum estrogen (E) (estrone (E_1. **9.3**) + estradiol (E_2. **9.1**)) concentration (-83.4) decreased together.

For simplicity, total serum estrogen (E) (estrone (E_1. **9.3**) + stradiol (E_2. **9.1**)) concentration and bioavailable serum estrogen (E) (estrone (E_1. **9.3**) + estradiol (E_2. **9.1**)) concentration were presented. However, estradiol (E_2. **9.1**) concentration and estrone (E_1. **9.3**)) concentration showed the similar change as total serum estrogen (E) (estrone (E_1. **9.3**) + stradiol (E_2. **9.1**)) concentration and bioavailable serum estrogen (E) (estrone (E_1. **9.3**) + estradiol (E_2. **9.1**)) concentration, respectively.

As expected from the beginning, there was a sharp drop in both total serum estrogen (E) (estrone (E_1. **9.3**) + stradiol (E_2. **9.1**)) concentration and bioavailable serum estrogen (E) (estrone (E_1. **9.3**) + estradiol (E_2. **9.1**)) concentration in women during menopause. On the other hand, there was a gradual, age-related decrease in bioavailable serum estrogen (E) (estrone (E_1. **9.3**) + estradiol (E_2. **9.1**)) concentration in the men.

There were also significant differences in the concentration change in serum sex hormone-binding globulin concentration (SHBG) with age. With regard to serum testosterone (T. **8.1**) concentration and serum estrogen (E) (estrone (E_1. **9.3**) + estradiol (E_2. **9.1**)) concentration between men and women, men have more than doubled their lifespan when compared to women T and E, but there was virtually no change in women.

Therefore, bioavailable reduction of serum testosterone (T. **8.1**) concentration in men and bioavailable large reduction of serum estrogen (E) (estrone (E_1. **9.3**) + estradiol (E_2. **9.1**)) concentration in women is that both of these decrease in the serum testosterone. T. **8.1**) concentration/sex hormone-binding globulin concentration (SHBG) (T/SHBG ratio) (log) and serum estrogen (E) (estrone (E_1. **9.3**) + estradiol (E_2. **9.1**))/sex hormone-binding globulin (SHBG) concentration (E/SHBG ratio) (log) may be due to the increase with age.

Then, as a result, serum dehydroepiandrosterone (DHEA. **7**) concentration also decreased significantly with age in both men and women.

In addition to the bioavailable sex steroid hormone, other bioavailable or free sex steroid hormone indices was investigated whether it decreased similarly with the age of men and women. Both age-related decrease in molar ratio of serum testosterone (T. **8.1**) concentration to serum sex hormone-binding globulin concentration (SHBG) and_serum estrogen (E) (estrone (E_1. **9.3**) + estradiol (E_2. **9.1**)) concentration to serum sex hormone-binding globulin concentration (SHBG) was almost similar to decrease in bioavailable serum testosterone (T. **8.1**) concentration and serum estrogen (E) (estrone (E_1. **9.3**) + estradiol (E_2. **9.1**)) concentration, respectively.

Furthermore, free serum testosterone. (T. **8.1**), which represents a fraction of serum testosterone (T. **8.1**) not bound to either serum sex hormone-binding globulin (SHBG) or albumin, decreased with age in a similar manner to bioavailable serum testosterone (T. **8.1**) concentrations in men and women.

The decrease in sex steroid hormones with age was a parallel increase in serum luteinizing hormone (LH) concentration and serum follicle-stimulating hormone (FSH) concentration.

Second, regarding the age-related changes in serum parathyroid hormone (PTH) and markers of bone turnover:

Change in excretion of serum parathyroid hormone (parathormone. PTH), an urinary protein secreted by osteoblasts osteocalcin (OC. **12**), and a degradation product of bone type I collagen and also a marker of osteoclast mediated bone resorption cross-linked *N*-telopeptide of type I collagen (NTx) in urine as a function of age for men and women was as follows [69]:

First, serum parathyroid hormone (parathormone. PTH) increased with age in men and women alike. During the life of men and women, the increase rate of serum parathyroid hormone (parathormone. PTH) was 84% in men and 64% in women, respectively.

Serum osteocalcin (OC. **12**) excretion and urinary cross-linked *N*-telopeptide of type I collagen (NTx) excretion decreased with age until around 50 years in men and then increased with age, respectively.

Like men, serum osteocalcin (OC. **12**) excretion and urinary cross-linked *N*-telopeptide of type I collagen (NTx) excretion in premenopausal women with age, increased with age in postmenopausal women.

Second, regarding the correlation coefficient (*r*) between markers of bone turnover and the age of men and women, serum bone-specific alkaline phosphatase (BAP) showed an age-related pattern similar to that of serum osteocalcin (OC. **12**). However, none of the individual correlation coefficients (*r*) showed statistical significance.

Third, serum carboxy-terminal propeptide of type I procollagen (PICP) decreased with age in men up to the age of 50 and in premenopausal women. Then, serum carboxy-terminal propeptide of type I procollagen

(PICP) showed little or no change with age in men over 50 or in postmenopausal women.

Fourth, the excretion of a collagen metabolite urinary free deoxypyridinoline (f-Dpd. **13**) (Figure 5) showed changes with age similar to urinary cross-linked *N*-telopeptide of type I collagen (NTx) excretion.

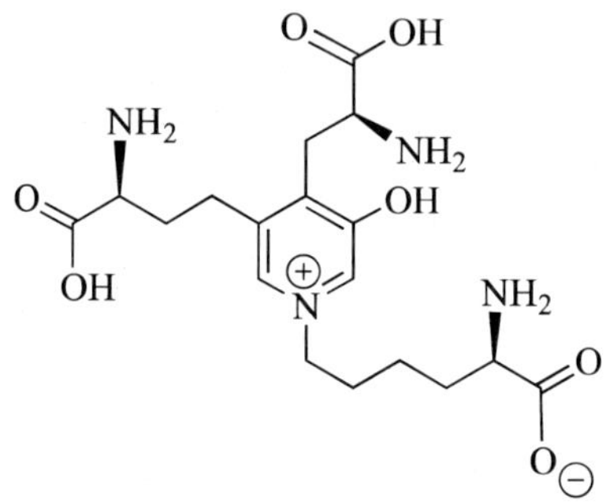

free deoxypyridinoline (f-Dpd. **13**)

Figure 5. Free deoxypyridinoline (f-Dpd. **13**).

Third, on relationship among bone mineral density (BMD), sex steroid hormone, and bone turnover.

First, according to the results of univariate analysis relating bone mineral density (BMD) at different skeletal sites for sex steroid hormone in men and women and dehydroepiandrosterone (DHEA. **7**) (Figure 3) concentration which is a kind of androgen produced in the adrenal and gonads, in men, total serum testosterone (T. **8.1**) concentration did not show relationship with bone mineral density (BMD) at any other site except for the weak part of the radius area. In contrast, bioavailable serum testosterone (T. **8.1**) concentration was correlated with bone mineral density (BMD) at all sites in men.

In women, serum testosterone (T. **8.1**) concentration and bioavailable serum testosterone (T. **8.1**) concentration showed the relationship equal to bone mineral density (BMD) at various sites.

Second, total bioavailable serum estrogen (E) (estrone (E_1. **9.3**) + estradiol (E_2. **9.1**)) concentrations correlated with bone mineral density (BMD) at various sites in men. However, the relationship between male total serum testosterone (T. **8.1**) and bone mineral density (BMD) showed higher bioavailability (BA) when compared to that (bioavailability (BA)) of total serum estrogen (E) (estrone (E_1. **9.3**) + estradiol (E_2. **9.1**)) concentration.

In contrast, total serum estrogen (E) (estrone (E_1. **9.3**) + estradiol (E_2. **9.1**)) concentration and bioavailable serum estrogen (E) (estrone (E_1. **9.3**) + estradiol (E_2. **9.1**)) concentration showed a similar relationship to bone mineral density (BMD) in women.

There was also a relationship between serum dehydroepiandrosterone sulfate (DHEA-S. **7'**) concentration and bone mineral density (BMD) in both men and women.

Third, from an univariate analysis associating bone mineral density (BMD at various sites in serum with serum parathyroid hormone (parathormone. PTH) and markers of bone turnover, serum parathyroid hormone (parathormone. PTH) showed inversely correlated with bone mineral density (BMD) at all sites in men and women except for total bone mineral density (BMD) in men.

All markers of bone turnover in men and women, except serum carboxy-terminal propeptide of type I procollagen (PICP), generally showed inverse correlation with bone mineral density (BMD) at various sites. However, the relationship between female markers of bone turnover and bone mineral density (BMD) was much higher when compared to that(relationship) of men.

Fourth, sex steroid hormones, especially bioavailable sex steroid hormone fraction, showed a marked inverse correlation with bone resorption markers.

From the first to third results above, older men showed a significant decrease in the concentration of bioavailable sex steroid hormon. This significant decrease showed a remarkable relationship with bone mineral density (BMD). In addition, the total bioavailable serum estrogen (E) (estrone. E_1 (**9.3**) + estradiol (E_2. **9.1**)) concentration predicts bone mineral density (BMD) of males and postmenopausal women. The concentration of bioavailable serum estrogen (E) (estrone (E_1. **9.3**) + estradiol (E_2. **9.1**)) suggests an important role in keletal metabolism of men and women.

In addition, there was a strikingly high relationship between serum parathyroid hormone (parathormone. PTH) and markers of bone turnover in elderly men and women. Combined with data from hormone receptor negative E-deficient and aromatase-deficient men [68, 70, 71, 72], it suggests the need to re-evaluate the traditional belief that the effects of sex steroid hormone concentrations on the skeleton of men is almost entirely due to the almost bioavailable serum testosterone (T. **8.1**)) concentration so far believed.

In the future, to compare the effects of bioavailable serum testosterone (T. **8.1**) and serum estrogen (E) (estrone (E_1. **9.3**) + estradiol (E_2. **9.1**)) concentrations on bone, additional longitudinal studies should be conducted. In addition, the hypothesis should be examined that calcium homeostasis in men and serum estrogen (E) (estrone (E_1. **9.3**) + estradiol (E_2. **9.1**)) concentration deficiency is the main cause of bone loss in elderly men [73].

CONCLUSION

For humans, various internal hormones are synthesized and secreted in specific organs such as growth hormone secreted from the pituitary gland in the body and parathyroid hormone secreted from the parathyroid gland, after that, circulates in the body through body fluids such as blood, and finally are essential physiologically active ingredients whicht exerts their physiological function effects on other specific cells. Hypersecretion of hormones or hyposecretion of hormones in humans can be one trigger that can cause serious dysfunction.

It has been suggested that supplementation with the eight typical hormones mentioned here is also effective for improving and curing hormone hyposecretion and so on. Based on these facts, hormonal therapy is expected to be safe for the body and to enhance the aging delay effect.

REFERENCES

[1] <https://ja.wikipedia.org/wiki/%E4%B8%8D%E8%80%81%E4%B8%8D%E6%AD%BB >.

[2] D'Costa AP, Ingram RL, Lenham JE, Sonntag WE. The regulation and mechanisms of action of growth hormone and insulin-like growth factor 1 during normal ageing. *J Reprod Fertil Suppl* 46, 87-98, 1993.

[3] Ho KY, Evans WS, Blizzard RM, Veldhuis JD, Merriam GR, Samojlik E, Furlanetto R, Rogol AD, Kaiser DL, Thorner MO. Effects of sex and age on the 24-hour profile of growth hormone secretion in man: importance of endogenous estradiol concentrations. *J Clin Endocrinol Metab* 64(1), 51-58, 1987.

[4] Frantz AG, Rabkin MT. Effects of estrogen and sex difference on secretion of human growth hormone. *J Clin Endocrinol Metab* 25(11), 1470-1480, 1965.

[5] Meistas MT, Foster GV, Margolis S, Kowarski AA Integrated concentrations of growth hormone, insulin, C-peptide and prolactin in human obesity. *Metabolism* 31(12), 1224-1228, 1982.

[6] Asplin CM, Faria AC, Carlsen EC, Vaccaro VA, Barr RE, Iranmanesh A, Lee MM, Veldhuis JD, Evans WS. Alterations in the pulsatile mode of growth hormone release in men and women with insulin-dependent diabetes mellitus. *J Clin Endocrinol Metab* 69(2), 239-245, 1989.

[7] Ho KY, Veldhuis JD, Johnson ML, Furlanetto R, Evans WS, Alberti KG, Thorner MO. Fasting enhances growth hormone secretion and amplifies the complex rhythms of growth hormone secretion in man. *J Clin Invest* 81(4), 968-975, 1988.

[8] Mauras N, Blizzard RM, Link K, Johnson ML, Rogol AD, Veldhuis JD. Augmentation of growth hormone secretion during puberty: evidence for a pulse amplitude-modulated phenomenon. *J Clin Endocrinol Metab* 64(3), 596-601, 1987.

[9] Zadik Z, Chalew SA, McCarter RJ Jr, Meistas M, Kowarski AA. The influence of age on the 24-hour integrated concentration of growth

hormone in normal individuals. *J Clin Endocrinol Metab* 60(3), 513-516, 1985.

[10] Finkelstein JW, Roffwarg HP, Boyar RM, Kream J, Hellman L Age-related change in the twenty-four-hour spontaneous secretion of growth hormone. *J Clin Endocrinol Metab* 35(5), 665-670, 1972.

[11] Carlson HE, Gillin JC, Gorden P, Snyder F. Absence of sleep-related growth hormone peaks in aged normal subjects and in acromegaly. *J Clin Endocrinol Metab* 34(6), 1102-1105, 1972.

[12] Rudman D, Kutner MH, Rogers CM, Lubin MF, Fleming GA, Bain RP. Impaired growth hormone secretion in the adult population: relation to age and adiposity. *J Clin Invest* 67(5), 1361-1369, 1981.

[13] Shibasaki T, Shizume K, Nakahara M, Masuda A, Jibiki K, Demura H, Wakabayashi I, Ling N. Age-related changes in plasma growth hormone response to growth hormone-releasing factor in man. *J Clin Endocrinol Metab* 58(1), 212-214, 1984.

[14] Prinz PN, Weitzman ED, Cunningham GR, Karacan I. Plasma growth hormone during sleep in young and aged men. *J Gerontol* 38(5), 519-524, 1983.

[15] Dudl RJ, Ensinck JW, Palmer HE, Williams RH. Effect of age on growth hormone secretion in man. *J Clin Endocrinol Metab* 37(1), 11-16, 1973.

[16] Florini JR, Prinz PN, Vitiello MV, Hintz RL. Somatomedin-C levels in healthy young and old men: relationship to peak and 24-hour integrated levels of growth hormone. *J Gerontol* 40(1), 2-7, 1985.

[17] Mauras N, Rogol AD, Veldhuis JD. Increased hGH production rate after low-dose estrogen therapy in prepubertal girls with Turner's syndrome. *Pediatr Res* 28(6), 626-630, 1990.

[18] Veldhuis JD, Iranmanesh A, Ho KK, Waters MJ, Johnson ML, Lizarralde G. Dual defects in pulsatile growth hormone secretion and clearance subserve the hyposomatotropism of obesity in man. *J Clin Endocrinol Metab* 72(1), 51-59, 1991.

[19] Hartman ML, Faria AC, Vance ML, Johnson ML, Thorner MO, Veldhuis JD. Temporal structure of *in vivo* growth hormone secretory events in humans. *Am J Physiol* 260(1 Pt 1), E101-E110, 1991.

[20] Veldhuis JD, Carlson ML, Johnson ML. The pituitary gland secretes in bursts: appraising the nature of glandular secretory impulses by simultaneous multiple-parameter deconvolution of plasma hormone concentrations. *Proc Natl Acad Sci USA* 84(21), 7686-7690, 1987.

[21] Iranmanesh A, Lizarralde G, Veldhuis JD. Age and relative adiposity are specific negative determinants of the frequency and amplitude of growth hormone (GH) secretory bursts and the half-life of endogenous GH in healthy men. *J Clin Endocrinol Metab* 73(5), 1081-1088, 1991.

[22] Tamarkin L, Baird CJ, Almeida OF. Melatonin: a coordinating signal for mammalian reproduction? *Science* 227(4688), 714-720, 1985.

[23] Wurtman JR, Waldhauser F (Eds). *Melatonin in Humans: Proceedings of the First International Conference on Melatonin in Humans* (*J Neural Transmission Supplementum*). 1986. Springer Verlag, NY, USA.

[24] Waldhauser F, Weiszenbacher G, Frisch H, Zeitlhuber U, Waldhauser M, Wurtman RJ. Fall in nocturnal serum melatonin during prepuberty and pubescence. *Lancet* 1(8373), 362-365, 1984.

[25] Gupta D, Riedel L, Frick HJ, Attanasio A, Ranke MB. Circulating melatonin in children: in relation to puberty, endocrine disorders, functional tests and racial origin. *Neuro Endocrinol Lett* 5(2), 63-78, 1983.

[26] Tamarkin L, Abastillas P, Chen HC, McNemar A, Sidbury JB. The daily profile of plasma melatonin in obese and Prader-Willi syndrome children. *J Clin Endocrinol Metab* 55(3), 491-495, 1982.

[27] Sizonenko PL, Lang U, Rivest RW, Aubert ML. The pineal and pubertal development. In: Evered D, Clark S (eds). *Photoperiodism, Melatonin and the Pineal*. Pitman, London, 208-230, 1985.

[28] Ehrenkranz JR, Tamarkin L, Comite F, Johnsonbaugh RE, Bybee DE, Loriaux DL, Cutler GB Jr. Daily rhythm of plasma melatonin in normal and precocious puberty. *J Clin Endocrinol Metab* 55(2), 307-310, 1982.

[29] Evered D, Clark S (eds). *Photoperiodism, melatonin and the pineal* (Ciba Foundation symposium). Distributed in North America by CIBA Pharmaceutical Co. (Medical Education Division), 1985. USA.
[30] Waldhauser F, Weiszenbacher G, Tatzer E, Gisinger B, Waldhauser M, Schemper M, Frisch H. Alterations in nocturnal serum melatonin levels in humans with growth and aging. *J Clin Endocrinol Metab* 66(3), 648-652, 1988.
[31] Wiener R, Utiger RD, Lew R, Emerson CH. Age, sex, and serum thyrotropin concentrations in primary hypothyroidism. *Acta Endocrinol (Copenh)* 124(4), 364-369, 1991.
[32] Hesch RD, Evered D. Radioimmunoassay of triiodothyronine in unextracted human serum. *Br Med J* 1(5854), 645-648, 1973.
[33] Gärtner R, Kewenig M, Horn K, Scriba PC. A new principle of thyroxine (T4) and triiodothyronine (T3) radioimmunoassay in unextracted serum using amisera with binding optima at extreme pH ranges. *J Clin Chem Clin Biochem* 18(9), 571-577, 1980.
[34] Gordon A, Gross J. An inter-laboratory comparison of total serum triiodothyronine determination. *Acta Endocrinol (Copenh)* 83(3), 539-548, 1976.
[35] Rubenstein HA, Butler VP Jr, Werner SC. Progressive decrease in serum triiodothyronine concentrations with human aging: radioimmunoassay following extraction of serum. *J Clin Endocrinol Metab* 37(2), 247-253, 1973.
[36] Hesch RD, Gatz J, Pape I, Sehmidt E, Mühlen AVZ: Total, free trüodothyronine and TBG concentration in elderly human persons. *Eur J Clin lnvest* 6, 139-145, 1976.
[37] Hesch RD, Emrich D, Mühlen AVZ, Breuel HP. Der Aussagewert der radioimmunchemischen Bestimmung von Trijodthyronin und thyreotropem Hormon rur die SchilddIÜsendiagnostik in der Praxis [The meaningfulness of the radioimmunochemical determination of triiodothyronine and thyroid hormone for thyroid diagnostics in practice]. *Dtsch Med Wschr* 100, 805-812, 1975.

[38] Hesch RD, Gatz J, Jüppner H, Stubbe P. TBG-dependency of age related variations of thyroxine and triiodothyronine. *Horm Metab Res* 9(2), 141-146, 1977.

[39] Heath H 3rd, Body JJ, Fox J. Radioimmunoassay of calcitonin in normal human plasma: problems, perspectives and prospects. *Biomed Pharmacother* 8(5), 241-245, 1984.

[40] Pedrazzoni M, Mantovani M, Ciotti G, Girasole G, Pioli G, Palummeri E. Calcitonin levels in normal women of various ages evaluated with a new sensitive radioimmunoassay. *Horm Metab Res* 20(2), 118-119, 1988.

[41] Hedge GA, Colby HD, Goodman RL. *Clinical Endocrine Physiology*, pp.127-159. 1987. W. B. Saunders Ltd., Philadelphia, USA.

[42] Schwartz AG, Pashko LL. Cancer prevention with dehydroepiandrosterone and non-androgenic structural analogs. *J Cell Biochem Suppl* 22, 210-217, 1995.

[43] Fettman MJ, Butler RN, McMichael AJ, Roberts-Thomson IC. Metabolic phenotypes and colorectal neoplasia. *J Gastroenterol Hepatol* 6(1), 81-89, 1991.

[44] Alberg AJ, Gordon GB, Hoffman SC, Comstock GW, Helzlsouer KJ. Serum dehydroepiandrosterone and dehydroepiandrosterone sulfate and the subsequent risk of developing colon cancer. *Cancer Epidemiol Biomarkers Prev* 9(5), 517-521, 2000.

[45] Orentreich N, Brind JL, Rizer RL, Vogelman JH. Age changes and sex differences in serum dehydroepiandrosterone sulfate concentrations throughout adulthood. *J Clin Endocrinol Metab* 59(3), 551-555, 1984.

[46] Bae CY, Lee SK, Lee YJ, Lee HT, Lee YG. Age changes and sex differences in serum dehydroepiandrosterone sulfate (DHEAS) concentrations & its related factors throughout adulthood. *J Korean Geriatr Soc* 2(2), 46-57, 1998.

[47] Nanba K, Vaidya A, Rainey WE. Aging and adrenal aldosterone production. *Hypertension* 71(2), 218-223, 2018.

[48] Hegstad R, Brown RD, Jiang NS, Kao P, Weinshilboum RM, Strong C, Wisgerhof M. Aging and aldosterone. *Am J Med* 74(3), 442-448, 1983.

[49] Lalli E, Barhanin J, Zennaro MC, Warth R. Local control of aldosterone production and primary aldosteronism. *Trends Endocrinol Metab* 27(3), 123-131, 2016.

[50] Nanba K, Vaidya A, Williams GH, Zheng I, Else T, Rainey WE. Age-related autonomous aldosteronism. *Circulation* 136(4), 347-355, 2017.

[51] Delmas PD, Stenner D, Wahner HW, Mann KG, Riggs BL. Increase in serum bone gamma-carboxyglutamic acid protein with aging in women. Implications for the mechanism of age-related bone loss. *J Clin Invest* 71(5), 1316-1321, 1983.

[52] Eastell R, Yergey AL, Vieira NE, Cedel SL, Kumar R, Riggs BL. Interrelationship among vitamin D metabolism, true calcium absorption, parathyroid function, and age in women: evidence of an age-related intestinal resistance to 1,25-dihydroxyvitamin D action. *J Bone Miner Res* 6(2), 125-132, 1991.

[53] Khosla S, Atkinson EJ, Melton LJ 3rd, Riggs BL. Effects of age and estrogen status on serum parathyroid hormone levels and biochemical markers of bone turnover in women: a population-based study. *J Clin Endocrinol Metab* 82(5), 1522-1527, 1997.

[54] McKane WR, Khosla S, Risteli J, Robins SP, Muhs JM, Riggs BL. Role of estrogen deficiency in pathogenesis of secondary hyperparathyroidism and increased bone resorption in elderly women. *Proc Assoc Am Physicians* 109(2), 174-180, 1997.

[55] Gallagher JC, Riggs BL, Eisman J, Hamstra A, Arnaud SB, DeLuca HF. Intestinal calcium absorption and serum vitamin D metabolites in normal subjects and osteoporotic patients: effect of age and dietary calcium. *J Clin Invest* 64(3), 729-736, 1979.

[56] Gennari C, Agnusdei D, Nardi P, Civitelli R. Estrogen preserves a normal intestinal responsiveness to 1,25-dihydroxyvitamin D3 in oophorectomized women. *J Clin Endocrinol Metab* 71(5), 1288-1293, 1990.

[57] Nordin BE, Need AG, Morris HA, Horowitz M, Robertson WG. Evidence for a renal calcium leak in postmenopausal women. *J Clin Endocrinol Metab* 72(2), 401-407, 1991.

[58] McKane WR, Khosla S, Burritt MF, Kao PC, Wilson DM, Ory SJ, Riggs BL. Mechanism of renal calcium conservation with estrogen replacement therapy in women in early postmenopause--a clinical research center study. *J Clin Endocrinol Metab* 80(12), 3458-3464, 1995.

[59] Cosman F, Nieves J, Horton J, Shen V, Lindsay R. Effects of estrogen on response to edetic acid infusion in postmenopausal osteoporotic women. *J Clin Endocrinol Metab* 78(4), 939-943, 1994.

[60] Riggs BL, Khosla S, Melton LJ 3rd. A unitary model for involutional osteoporosis: estrogen deficiency causes both type I and type II osteoporosis in postmenopausal women and contributes to bone loss in aging men. *J Bone Miner Res* 13(5), 763-773, 1998.

[61] Harman SM, Tsitouras PD. Reproductive hormones in aging men. I. Measurement of sex steroids, basal luteinizing hormone, and Leydig cell response to human chorionic gonadotropin. *J Clin Endocrinol Metab* 51(1), 35-40, 1980.

[62] Foresta C, Ruzza G, Mioni R, Guarneri G, Gribaldo R, Meneghello A, Mastrogiacomo I. Osteoporosis and decline of gonadal function in the elderly male. *Horm Res* 19(1), 18-22, 1984.

[63] Meier DE, Orwoll ES, Keenan EJ, Fagerstrom RM. Marked decline in trabecular bone mineral content in healthy men with age: lack of association with sex steroid levels. *J Am Geriatr S*oc 35(3), 189-197, 1987.

[64] Riggs BL, Wahner HW, Dunn WL, Mazess RB, Offord KP, Melton LJ 3rd. Differential changes in bone mineral density of the appendicular and axial skeleton with aging: relationship to spinal osteoporosis. *J Clin Invest* 67(2), 328-335, 1981.

[65] Jones G, Nguyen T, Sambrook P, Kelly PJ, Eisman JA. Progressive loss of bone in the femoral neck in elderly people: longitudinal findings from the Dubbo osteoporosis epidemiology study. *BMJ* 309(6956), 691-695, 1994.

[66] Murphy S, Khaw KT, Cassidy A, Compston JE. Sex hormones and bone mineral density in elderly men. *Bone Miner* 20(2), 133-140, 1993.

[67] Slemenda CW, Longcope C, Zhou L, Hui SL, Peacock M, Johnston CC. Sex steroids and bone mass in older men. Positive associations with serum estrogens and negative associations with androgens. *J Clin Invest* 100(7), 1755-1759, 1997.

[68] Smith EP, Boyd J, Frank GR, Takahashi H, Cohen RM, Specker B, Williams TC, Lubahn DB, Korach KS. Estrogen resistance caused by a mutation in the estrogen-receptor gene in a man. *N Engl J Med* 331(16), 1056-1061, 1994.

[69] von Schewelov T, Carlsson A, Dahlberg L. Cross-linked *N*-telopeptide of type I collagen (NTx) in urine as a predictor of periprosthetic osteolysis. *J Orthop Res* 24(7), 1342-1348, 2006.

[70] Morishima A, Grumbach MM, Simpson ER, Fisher C, Qin K. Aromatase deficiency in male and female siblings caused by a novel mutation and the physiological role of estrogens. *J Clin Endocrinol Metab* 80(12), 3689-3698, 1995.

[71] Carani C, Qin K, Simoni M, Faustini-Fustini M, Serpente S, Boyd J, Korach KS, Simpson ER. Effect of testosterone and estradiol in a man with aromatase deficiency. *N Engl J Med* 337(2), 91-95, 1997.

[72] Morishima A, Grumbach MM, Bilezikian JP. Estrogen markedly increases bone mass in an estrogen deficient young man with aromatase deficiency. *J Bone Miner Res* 12(Suppl 1), S126, 1977.

[73] Khosla S, Melton LJ 3rd, Atkinson EJ, O'Fallon WM, Klee GG, Riggs BL. Relationship of serum sex steroid levels and bone turnover markers with bone mineral density in men and women: a key role for bioavailable estrogen. *J Clin Endocrinol Metab* 83(7), 2266-2274, 1998.

ABOUT THE EDITOR

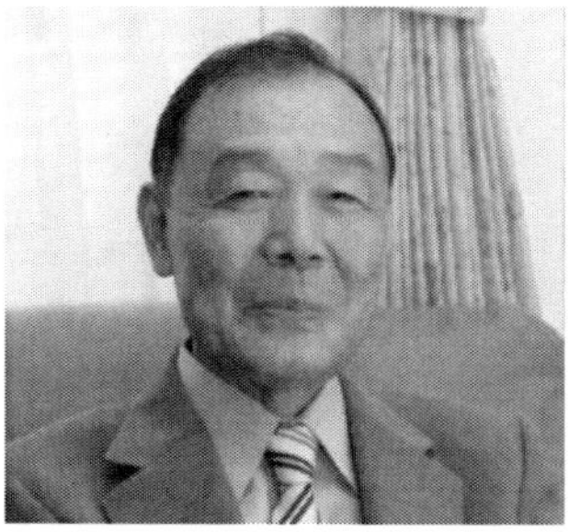

Noboru Motohashi

Foreign examiner for evaluation of the Ph.D. thesis in Indian National University, India; Former Professor and Director (elected Riji in Japanese) of *Meiji Pharmaceutical University*, Tokyo, Japan

E-mail: noborumotohashi@jcom.home.ne.jp

Professional Appointments:

1966: Pharmaceutical Sciences, *Tohoku University*, Sendai, Japan (graduated school)

1985-1986: Visiting Professor of Department of Medicinal Chemistry, College of Pharmacy, *Univesity of Kansas (KU)*, Lawrence, KS, USA

2006: Professor of *Meiji Pharmaceutical University*, Tokyo, Japan (retired)

2007: Advisor of *Meiji Pharmaceutical University*, Tokyo, Japan (retired)

2011: Elected Director (Riji in Japanese) of *Meiji Pharmaceutical University*, Tokyo, Japan (retired).

INDEX

A

D

E

I

L

M

N

O

U

V

W

Y